Table of Contents

INTRODUCTION

You may or may not have heard of intermittent fasting. It is a fairly simple nutritional intervention that is widespread. You have to split your 24-hour day into two basic states or categories.

"Fast" -ed or "Fast" -ing condition: (Between 18 and 48 hours)

"Fed" or "feed" status

The Word Web Dictionary shows that the word "intermittent" means "stop and start at irregular intervals." That is, when it comes to fasting, do not fast daily or for long periods. Eat for a few days. After fasting for one day, eat again. In fact, this is the only healthy way to lose weight on an empty stomach and works well if done correctly. Performing incorrectly can cause real problems. Yes, fasting and weight loss work well together and have many great benefits:

- You don't have to buy special food.

- You can eat the foods you love.

- There are no complicated rules to follow.

- It's cheap to do ... don't buy special foods.

- It is fun.

- You can stay on this type of weight loss system for a lifetime.

The body was designed to feed on fat when there was no food available. If the family hunter has caught something that he has eaten for a few days, he has to catch something else. If you looked at pictures of people 100 years ago (when it was more difficult to get food), you will notice very few fat people. Our constant access to food has really caused a big problem in our country. Even our children are overweight and suffer from health problems. Intermittent fasting is normal, healthy, and pleasant ... and the best thing is that it is great for losing weight. Let's look at your fasting state first. The time ranges from 16 to 48 hours. To begin with, you usually have dinner at 7 or 8 pm. In this example, you then enter your fast for the next 16 to 18 hours. You would then wake up the next morning and possibly complete your morning workout or prepare for work. You would then try to consume your first meal between 11 am and 1 pm that day. Things to keep in mind while fasting:

Possible irritability

Increased need for water consumption

Greater ability to distinguish between false and real hunger

Large calorie deficit and reset of the hormonal environment of the body's fat-burning.

Intermittent fasting (IF) refers to eating habits where no calories are eaten for a long period of time or calories are severely restricted. Fasting or periods of voluntary abstention from food have been practiced around the world for centuries. Intermittent fasting with the aim of improving health relatively new. Intermittent fasting involves restricting food intake for a set period of time and does not involve changes to the actual foods you eat. Currently, the main IF protocols are a 16-hour daily fast and a full day, one or two days a week fast. Intermittent fasting could be seen as a natural eating pattern that man was made to do, and goes back to our Paleolithic ancestors of hunters and gatherers. Current models of planned intermittent fasting programs have the potential to improve many aspects of health, from body composition to longevity and aging. Although IFviolates the norms of our culture and general daily routines, science may suggest a lower frequency of meals and more fasting as an optimal alternative to the normal breakfast, lunch, and dinner model. Intermittent fasting has many different subgroups, each with individual fluctuations in the duration of fasting, some hours, and other days. This has become a prevalent topic in science due to the potential health and fitness benefits being discovered. Here are two common myths related to intermittent fasting.

Myth 1-1 Need to eat three meals a day: This "rule" common in Western societies is not developed based on evidence of improved health but adopted as a general pattern of settlers And eventually became the norm. Not only does the three-meal-day model lack scientific justification, but recent studies have shown that reducing food and increasing fasting is optimal for human health. One study showed that once-daily meals with the same amount of daily calories in weight loss and body composition were better than three times daily meals. This finding is a basic concept that extrapolates to intermittent fasting, and those who choose IF may find it best to eat only 1-2 meals a day.

Myth 2 - You need breakfast, it's the prevalent meal of the day: Many false claims have been made about the absolute need for daily breakfast. The most common claims are "breakfast increases metabolism" and "breakfast decreases food intake later in the day." These claims were refuted and investigated over a 16 week period. The results showed that skipping breakfast did not decrease metabolism and did not increase food intake at lunch and dinner. It is still possible to make intermittent fasting logs while having breakfast, but some people find it easier to eat a late breakfast or to skip it entirely, and this common myth shouldn't be in the way.

The eating pattern called "intermittent fasting" usually means fasting for a while and eating for a while. Many choose a 24-hour fasting cycle, then eat healthy the next day and continue this process as a lifestyle change. Studies have been done on animals to find out the benefits of this type of fasting, and you will be happy to know that this can be really beneficial to your health! Intermittent fasting can extend your life by 40% to 56%! That alone is reason enough to do it. However, other benefits include weight loss and fat oxidation. When you fast, your body has to search for fuel, which will remove aged and damaged cells. This type of cleansing cleanses the body of unwanted and unwanted things and helps increase weight loss and the benefits of good food choices and brings more benefits to your body. It has been shown that rats with heart failure have long-term and improved survival even after an IF diet. Researchers also say that it could also help age-related cognitive deficits. Your risk of heart disease and other heart conditions may also be reduced if you start healthy intermittent fasting. Your risk of other chronic diseases will most likely also be reduced.

The healthier you can start with intermittent fasting and a healthy selection of foods! Keep carbohydrates at 50-100 grams a day. Many women eat between 1200 and 1500 calories a day, and if they limit their carbohydrates, they still lose weight. Men can handle up to 2000 calories a day. Of course, less is best, and you need to measure calories based on your activities, such as Determine hard work and exercise. Drink plenty of fluids, especially water, and exercise in the evening if possible. This will help with these nightly desires. As soon as you start eating and drinking healthier, your body no longer craves (if at all) junk food, so choosing healthy foods becomes easier as you go on intermittent fasting. Alternative daytime fasting or ADF means alternating eating and not eating, but there is also intermittent fasting called Modified Fasting, in which you consume about 20% of your normal calories one day and eat normal (but healthy) the next day. This is often more achievable for people because they feel less disadvantaged if they can eat at least daily, and it still has most of the benefits of the ADF regime. Whatever you do, make sure you tell your doctor about your plans so that he or she is aware of it and can work with you to achieve your goals. If you want to lose weight, lose fat, and feel better, intermittent fasting may be the answer for you!

Intermittent fasting includes alternating periods of feasts and hunger, during which you can eat as much as you want during the festival, but only drink water during fasting. The goal is to take advantage of calorie reduction and use it as a weight-loss vehicle for some. Intermittent fasting can take place over several days, alternating between 24 hours and daily. The first option requires you to skip some or all meals on one or more days of the week. Daily fasting includes 24-hour periods of eating and fasting that end at the same time each day, e.g., For example, eat as much as you like from Monday 6 pm to Tuesday 6 pm, Tuesday 6 pm to Wednesday 6 pm and repeat the process. During daily intermittent fasting, there is short mealtime, usually 4-6 hours within the 24-hour day, in which you can consume as much as you like. Some of the things that scare people away are the fear that they are extremely hungry and do not stick to the schedule or do not know how to include it in their schedule. This is actually quite simple if you plan in advance that you will eat your dinner almost every day at the same time, but at an hour on both sides, depending on whether it is an intermittent fasting or eating phase. With a little planning, you can also make contacts and eat out here. The main reason preventing many people from trying is the fear of being hungry. Although this requires a little willpower and a little discomfort, it's actually quite simple!

Types Of Intermittent Fasting

Intermittent fasting comes in several forms, and each can have a number of specific advantages. Every form of intermittent fasting shows variations in the ratio of fasting to eating. The benefits and effectiveness of these different protocols can vary individually, and it is important to determine which one is best for you. The factors that can influence the selection include health goals, daily routine/routine, and current state of health. The most common types of IF are second-day fasting, temporary feeding, and modified fasting.

1. FASTING ON THE ALTERNATIVE DAY:

This approach alternates between days without calories (from food or drinks) with days of free feeding and eating whatever you want. This plan has been shown to help you lose weight, improve blood cholesterol and triglyceride (fat) levels, and improve blood inflammation markers. The main disadvantage of this form of intermittent fasting is that due to the reported hunger during fasting days, it is the most difficult to stick to.

2. CHANGED FAST - 5: 2 DIET

Modified fasting is a protocol with programmed fasting days, but the fasting days allow some food intake. In general, 20-25% of normal calories can be consumed on fasting days. So if you normally consume 2000 calories on normal eating days, you can consume 400-500 calories on fasting days. The 5: 2 part of this diet relates to the ratio of non-fasting to fasting days. With this regime, you would normally eat for 5 consecutive days and then reduce the calorie count to 20-25% for 2 consecutive days. This protocol is ideal for weight loss and body composition and can also help regulate blood sugar, lipids, and inflammation. Studies have shown that the 5: 2 protocol for weight loss is effective, improves/lowers inflammation markers in the blood, and shows signs of an improvement in insulin resistance. In animal studies, this modified 5: 2 fasting diet resulted in a reduction in fat, a decrease in hunger hormones (leptin), and an increased protein level, which is responsible for the improvement in fat burning and blood sugar regulation (adiponectin). The modified 5: 2 fasting protocol is easy to follow and has a small number of negative side effects, including hunger, low energy, and some irritability at the start of the program. In contrast, studies have also found improvements such as reduced tension, less anger, less fatigue, improvement in self-confidence, and a more positive mood.

3. TIME-LIMITED FEEDING:

If you know someone who has said that they are fasting temporarily, the chances are that it is a temporary feed. This kind of intermittent fasting is used daily, consumes only a few calories of the day, and fasts the rest. The daily fasting intervals with time-limited feeding can be between 12 and 20 hours, the most common method being 16/8 (16 hours of fasting, consuming 8 calories). In this protocol, time is not important as long as you fast for consecutive hours and eat only the time allowed. For example, in a limited time 16/8 feeding program, one person may eat the first meal around 7 am and the last meal at 3 pm. (From 3:00 pm to 7:00 am), others can eat the first meal at 1:00 pm. Last meal at 9:00 pm (fast from 9:00 am to 1:00 pm). This protocol is intended to run for a long time every day and is very flexible during fasting/meal times. Time-limited feeding is one of the easiest to follow intermittent fasting methods. If you use this together with your daily work and sleep schedule, you can achieve an optimal metabolic function. Time-limited feeding is a great program for improving weight loss and body composition, as well as some other general health benefits. A small number of human studies conducted have shown significant weight loss, fasting blood sugar, and improved cholesterol without altering perceived tension, depression, anger, fatigue, or confusion. Some other preliminary results from animal studies showed temporary feeding to protect against obesity, high insulin levels, fatty liver disease, and inflammation. Ease of use and the promising results of temporary feeding could potentially make it an excellent option for weight loss and chronic disease prevention/treatment. When implementing this protocol, it may make sense to start with lower fasting to eating ratio, such as 12/12 hours, and then work your way up to 16/8 hours.

Intermittent fasting is a particularly interesting option compared to other nutritional approaches. Does an intermittent fasting diet work compare to other diets? The answer here is a resounding yes. For example, if you fast for 16 hours, your body burns fat almost every day! And if you get all of your calories during a relatively small meal window, your body can't go into hunger mode and desperately cling to body fat. Compared to a normal low-calorie diet, this is a big difference. While any low-calorie approach initially leads to fat loss, your body is an efficient machine and balances it out by slowing down your metabolism (exactly the opposite of what you want) and holding on to body fat. Is intermittent fasting restrictive? Every diet inherently includes a better selection of foods. If someone tries to sell you the pancake diet, walk a mile! Eating garbage can never be a good choice. With most diets, however, you have to try to eat clean all the time. This is very difficult to do and is directly related to eating 12 donuts in one session after a few weeks of withdrawal! Intermittent fasting also includes a healthy selection of foods, but it gives you more leeway. It is difficult to eat too much garbage in a small meal window after you have already eaten healthily. However, you can eat enough to prevent yourself from falling off the cart. Perhaps the real benefit of intermittent fasting is that it can be a lifestyle rather than a short-term approach. Even if you manage to stick to most diets long enough to get results, there is usually a rebound, a return to poor eating, and fat gain. If you consider fasting as a long-term solution, this problem effectively disappears.

HEALTH BENEFITS OF INTERMITTENT FASTING

This process of natural cleansing enables the body to remove harmful toxins from the body. People who lose unwanted body fat and want to build the desired muscles tend to adjust a fasting program. Burning fat while exercising in a ketogenic state is one of the preferred routines for weight loss. For many people, fasting improves not only their physical health but also their general well-being. Their energy level is more stable, and they are generally in a better mood. Fasting improves mental focus and general concentration. The stimulating hormone catecholamine is released in abundance during Lent. As a result, there is increased mental focus and productivity, and a general feeling of satisfaction with everything you do.

Intermittent fasting or IF for short is not a dietary or hungry process—eating pattern. Fasting and reducing calorie intake will make you healthier and longer. Our ancestors were our former collectors and hunters. They weren't always eating, and what they ate was based on what was available. If this is said, it means that our body is actually designed to stay without food for hours. You can survive without eating three meals a day, and living IF life has many benefits.

You keep yourself full. Some people think that fasting or dieting is hungry for the matter. However, when intermittent fasting is done, ghrelin, a hormone that signals hunger, adapts to the new way of eating the body, which is why you won't feel hungry.

You have better focus and concentration. Fasting produces more catecholamines, another hormone in the body. So the bottom line is that you focus more on what you're doing.

You will have more energy. Because you don't eat that much, your blood sugar level fluctuates less. This means that the real energy is evener. They also reduce the risk of developing diabetes. You can also exercise while on the go, which increases your body's potential to burn more fats. A growth hormone increases when you fast, which helps burn calories.

You burn more fat, which means weight loss. Because you eat less and eat fewer calories, your body turns into body fat to burn energy instead of taking the energy from the food that is otherwise eaten regularly if you do not fast intermittently. This also means that your body shows more bouts of muscle mass. By the way, if you fast for about 16 hours, your body is already consuming body fat.

You can also benefit from Less blood glucose and better insulin levels.

Psychological and health benefits. In addition to the benefit of a quick reduction in body fat, there are other less obvious but important reasons why intermittent fasting is good long-term health and fat loss plan. From a health point of view, your system is cleaned at any speed because your body gets used to the fact that less food is added. This has a lot to do with taking control of food, appetite, and the little triggers that drove much of my food. When you clearly recognize this and regain control, you can break the cycle and start to introduce more positive eating habits into your life. This is very important to manage your weight and health not only in the short term but also for the rest of your life. I am a firm supporter of intermittent fasting as a way to fast, healthy weight loss. If you are serious about wanting a lean, healthy body for life, I strongly recommend that you think about trying it.

Intermittent fasting cleanses your inner body. Just as you would have to clean your outer body of dirt, you must also clean the inside of chemicals and other harmful substances from your food intake. It removes toxins that may have accumulated in your colon, making you feel healthier and avoiding a variety of potential health risks.

When your body is free of toxic substances, your digestive and other systems work optimally. You will experience better digestion because your body uses the food you eat more efficiently. Better use of food means that you no longer feel the need to eat unnecessarily, and if you remove all excess food, your body will naturally stop gaining weight.

Intermittent fasting is a phenomenon these days. Recent studies have shown that those who try to lose weight, improve health, and have a longer lifespan. In other words, a person can eat whatever they want within 24 hours and fast for the next 24 hours. This approach to weight control appears to be supported by science as well as religious and cultural practices around the world. Intermittent fasters claim that this practice is a way to be more careful with food. There are many different popular intermittent fasting and hundreds of other possible variations. There are two kinds of intermittent fasting that are the easiest and most commonly used. The first is daily fasting, in which the person is only allowed to eat once every 20 to 28 hours within 4 hours. The second is fasting for 1-3 times a week, also called fasting on the second day, in which a person eats everything he wants in one day and fasts the next day. Intermittent fasting has many beneficial effects as it has been tested on animals such as rodents and primates. One study found that there was "decreased serum glucose and insulin levels and increased neuron resistance in the brain to excitotoxicity stress."

Your body does not try to hold onto its fat reserves during intermittent fasting. Most nutritional approaches are necessarily restrictive. Enough food is constantly being withdrawn from your body, and it reacts to going into hunger mode. It depends on all of your fat reserves and slows down your metabolism, just the opposite of what we want. However, if you can eat to your satisfaction like a fast-food diet, your body responds by continuing to reduce body fat. An intermittent fasting diet is less restrictive than other diets. Let us be clear here, if your idea of good food is a burger and fries, nothing will help you until you change your perception. However, it is quite possible and even helpful to have some leeway when eating. Sure, start with your protein and vegetables, but some of what you like has some interesting and positive hormonal effects when you try to slim down or even build muscle. An intermittent fasting diet adapts to you. This is the real beauty of this approach. Instead of finding exactly the right number of grams of carbohydrates or whatever at 10 am, adjust your daily fast to your life and goals. Some find that a 16-hour fast works best from noon to noon the next day. Others prefer a 24-hour cycle or even a 4-hour meal window. All of this is possible and has different advantages. It's more of a lifestyle than a diet. It may be hard to believe, but intermittent fasting has huge benefits. The main thing is that many important parts and organs of your body rest so that they can do their job better. Some of them are:

* Increased insulin sensitivity/nutrient portioning is a great way to build muscle without gaining fat!

* Increased adrenaline/noradrenaline, which means that more time is spent burning fat!

* Reduced appetite and hunger, possibility to feel full because all calories are eaten in fewer meals

* Increased energy and concentration

*Lowering the level of glucose

* Increase in growth hormone

* Burning fat

*Increase glucagon (helps burn fat)

*Reduce inflammation. The digestive system rests; this, in turn, helps many other parts of the body.

*It reduces blood sugar. This reduces insulin production and makes it more sensitive and effective. It also rests the pancreas.

*High blood pressure is checked.

*Detoxification takes place. Fasting helps cleanse and detoxify your body. It is important to drink plenty of water for this.

*It increases your energy and makes you feel better.

*It protects you from heart disease and strokes.

*It helps to strengthen your immune system and thus fights excessive (chronic) inflammation.

*It reduces oxidative stress caused by free radicals in your cells.

Some surprising and different advantages

The most obvious benefits include lowering high blood pressure, checking diabetes, longer lifespan, lowering stress levels, and a feel-good factor, as well as significant weight loss in a short amount of time. When you start such a fasting program, make sure you start slowly, e.g., For example, fast one day a week until your body is ready to accept a two-day fast. During this time, design your bodyweight training plans appropriately, preferably at a moderate pace, until your body is able to perform a fully loaded workout routine. When you get used to it, the results show positive on your body. If you're looking for exercise and diet options that promise to get significant results in a short amount of time, try intermittent fasting as an effective solution. However, intermittent fasting gives your body a little boost with the fat burning function. Your body will suddenly learn how to burn a lot of fat in a short time. Intermittent refers to fasting; do not eat anything and only drink water for at least 24 hours. As unbelievable as this may seem, intermittent fasting has been very successful for many people in helping them lose weight and generally feel better. Intermittent fasting helps our body burn fat quickly in a variety of ways.

It is a program where you fast once or twice a week. So you only use water twice a week. This method can cause you to lose a lot of weight quickly, and it is not unhealthy despite popular belief. Think about how to lose weight. It's easy; you just have to consume more calories than you consume. If you go without calories 2 full days a week, you will dramatically speed up your weight loss process. One thing that may worry you is that you don't have enough energy to continue your exercise program. Well, that's only the case if you're permanently fasting on consecutive days. With intermittent fasting, you only fast once every few days, so you still have the energy to complete your workout. In fact, it actually helps speed up your metabolism and can actually increase your energy level.

Another advantage of fasting is that it cleanses your body. If you only drink water for a whole day, you will remove all the toxins in your body from your normal diet. If you get rid of these toxins, you can lose weight faster and feel better when fasting. Try intermittent fasting when trying to lose weight. Start by doing very moderate exercises only once a week. If you think you can control it, start strengthening and have a regular exercise program until you do it twice a week.

It can also help mitigate the risk of chronic diseases such as diabetes, cancer, and heart disease. Intermittent fasting is really nothing new. In fact, IF goes far back to our original ancestors. It is an eating strategy imprinted on our DNA because our ancestors practiced a reduced eating plan. They literally had no choice. They just didn't have the frequency and easy access to the food we have now.

This new eating strategy is not just about skipping meals. Spend as much time as possible in a fasted state. The better option to define any type of fasting is to simply consider dietary changes. In the case of IF, instead of three square meals in a day or eating a handful of smaller meals during the day, there is a time window in which we are allowed to eat. This can take a few hours a day, or the fasting window can represent certain days of the week. During this time, we can eat what we want - of course, within reason.

When we leave our "eating window," our minds can adjust to our bodies so that we understand what real hunger really feels like. IF it's not about starvation, fasting does not mean starving, but it is also not a diet. The literal definition is: "to refrain from eating and drinking for a certain period of time."

IF it's about eating two meals in a day instead of three (or more) during which you introduce a 16-hour fast. IF doesn't work for someone whose diet focuses on processed foods like chips. When fasting, the main thing we need to do is to eat whole foods that are rich in vegetables, lean protein, healthy carbohydrates, and fats to get the best and fastest benefits from IF. The two meals selected for the day must be packed in a nutritious and balanced manner. It is evaluated that one in two people in today's modern world is obese or overweight, and millions die from complications arising from this truth. Intermittent fasting helps to manage body weight and is also a powerful tool in the area of life extension.

If you don't eat late into the night, you are likely already adding some form of IF to your schedule and fasting for about 12 hours a day. However, recent research shows that some benefits of IF require longer periods of fasting, depending on the level of activity, up to 20 to 24 hours. The proposed benefits of Intermittent fasting in animals and humans read like a laundry list of "looking better," "feeling better," and "living longer" ... Having a restricted eating window is much less difficult than restricting calories. IF is actually one of the easiest strategies for losing fat and maintaining good weight (muscle tissue) and requires few changes in behavior. Slowing down the aging process, raising energy levels, and restarting the immune system are the benefits of including IF in your diet. What are you looking to Decide which two meals you want to enjoy in the future and choose the richest and nutritious food you want to enjoy in the meantime. Following this protocol, when combined with challenging strength training exercises, you will see positive changes in body and feel.

The benefits of fasting are great news these days. But how effective is it? Most people are interested in it as a weight-loss tool, and in fact, you can use it to lose weight, but in fact, there are many benefits beyond weight loss, some of which are very miraculous. It has long been known to significantly extend the life of mice, worms, and flies, and even extend the life of monkeys. Does it prolong human life? Many people are convinced of this, but the truth is that although it looks hopeful, we are still not sure. However, there is no doubt that it has health benefits related to heart disease, cancer, dementia, and even your mood and well-being. Although not a cure, it creates a condition for healing by resting and restoring important parts of the body. There is no doubt that overeating is stressful on your body and that it occasionally needs a break. Indeed, studies have shown that when it is not at rest, it does without much of the repair and regeneration necessary for optimal health.

Less Inflammation

Protection against diseases such as heart disease, Alzheimer's, and cancer. Increases metabolism, which leads to weight and body fat loss. Unlike a daily calorie reduction diet, intermittent fasting increases your metabolism. This makes sense from a survival perspective. When we are not eating, the body uses stored energy as fuel so that we can stay alive to find another meal. Hormones enable the body to switch energy sources from food to body fat. Studies clearly show this phenomenon. For example, a 4-day fast increased basal metabolic rate by 12%. The level of the neurotransmitter norepinephrine, which prepares the body for the action, rose by 117%. The fatty acids in the bloodstream increased by over 370% as the body switched from burning food to burning stored fat.No loss of muscle mass unlike a constant calorie diet, intermittent fasting does not burn the muscles, as many feared. In 2010, the researchers examined a group of subjects who were fasted alternately daily for 70 days (ate one day and fasted the next). Their muscle mass started at 52.0 kg and ended at 51.9 kg. In other words, there was no muscle loss, but 11.4% fat was lost, and LDL cholesterol and triglyceride levels improved significantly. During fasting, the body naturally develops more human growth hormone and maintains lean muscle and bone. Muscle mass is generally retained until body fat drops below 4%. Therefore, for most people, intermittent fasting poses no risk of muscle wasting.

Type 2 diabetes is a disease in which there is simply too much sugar in the body so that the cells no longer respond to insulin and can absorb more glucose from the blood (insulin resistance), which leads to high blood sugar. The liver is also loaded with fat when it tries to get rid of the excess glucose by converting it to fat and storing it as fat. To reverse this situation, you need to do two things: First, avoid giving your body more sugar. Second, burn the remaining sugar. The best diet to meet this is a low carb, low protein, high-fat diet, also known as a ketone diet. (Remember that carbohydrates increase blood sugar the most, protein to a certain extent, and fat the least.) For this reason, a low-carbohydrate diet helps reduce exposure to incoming glucose. For some people, this is enough to reverse insulin resistance and type 2 diabetes. In more severe cases, however, a diet alone is not enough. Exercise helps burn glucose in the skeletal muscles, but not in all tissues and organs, including fatty liver. Of course, exercise is important, but in order to get rid of the excess glucose in the organs, the cells have to "starve" temporarily. This can be achieved by intermittent fasting. For this reason, historically, fasting has been called cleansing or detoxification. It becomes a very powerful tool to get rid of all excesses. This is the fastest way to lower blood sugar and insulin levels and eventually reverse insulin resistance, fatty liver, and type 2 diabetes. Moreover, taking insulin for type 2 diabetes does not correct the main cause of the problem: the excess sugar in the body. It's true that insulin drives the blood sugar out of the blood to lower it, but where does sugar go? The liver will simply turn everything into fat, fat in the liver, and fat in the stomach. Patients who take insulin often gain weight, making their diabetes worse.

Improve heart health-Over time, hyperglycemia from type 2 diabetes can damage the blood vessels and nerves that control the heart. The longer diabetes, the more likely it is to develop heart disease. Lowering blood sugar through intermittent fasting also reduces the risk of cardiovascular disease and stroke. IF has also been shown to improve blood pressure, total and LDL cholesterol (bad cholesterol), blood triglycerides, and inflammation markers associated with many chronic diseases.

Increases brain performance - Several studies have shown that fasting has many neurological benefits, including attention and focus, response time, immediate memory, cognition, and new brain cell production. IF reduces brain inflammation and prevents the symptoms of Alzheimer's.

Improve Clarity

Regardless of whether you want to lose the much-needed weight or just want to clean your system, intermittent fasting has many benefits for the body. The first thing you need to clarify is that fasting is NOT the same as starving. Yes, while it is true that fasting means not eating, intermittent fasting is gradually being done. Fasting is a completely natural part of life and has been practiced for one reason or another for millions of years. Fasting is used in many successful diet programs today. People become overweight if they consume more calories than they burn at the same time. With the sedentary lifestyle that many of us have, this has become very common. Fortunately, there are much great fitness, weight loss, and exercise programs to solve the overweight problem. Unfortunately, many cannot afford or find the time to integrate them into their busy lifestyle. Intermittent fasting can be very helpful for those people who want to lose weight. Regardless of what we do regularly, it's always good to just take a day off. The same goes for food. Many junk and harmful toxins enter our bodies every day. By taking a day off (intermittent fasting), we give our body the opportunity to get rid of these harmful and unnecessary things. Drinking plenty of water while fasting will make it easier and help cleanse the body. People who practice intermittent fasting have found that they feel healthier and have better health overall. Intermittent fasting has many benefits for the body, the first of which is to empty the body for a day without anything returning to it. Second, your body will experience improved insulin resistance, which plays a big role in many functions, including better performance, muscle gain, weight loss, disease prevention, anti-aging, and just a better immune system in general. If the idea of fasting is scary to you, you will quickly change your mind when you see the many benefits it offers to your body and overall health. There is no way to fast intermittently. As with everything new, you need to do what works best for your lifestyle and personal habits. Make IF a part of your life, and you will soon see the benefits. The first is that you feel better. As you fast for a day, detoxify and cleanse your body without replacing the things you want to get rid of. It is a win-win situation for your body.

Intermittent fasting is a very important factor in any fat loss plan, and you need to include it in your workout to get better results. Fasting is the process of only drinking water and not having to eat for 24 hours. In the process, both your fat and your weight loss. This process reduces your daily calorie intake and still adheres to a complete exercise plan. Fasting is a very good tool for those who are really serious about fat loss and muscle building.

The main reason why you should do this is that intermittent fasting consumes maximum fats. Imagine if you only fast two days a week, you reduce a whole full calorie quota of two days from your weekly consumption! Combined with your daily workout, you can get great results and lose excess fat.

The second reason for fasting is that you can maintain a moderate to intense exercise load without losing your energy and metabolism. Most people think that fasting drains your energy and metabolism, but that's not true. Adding fasting to your diet will give you more energy and metabolism.

The third reason why fasting is good practice to include in your training plan is its beneficial aspects that bring you great benefits. If you do any kind of fasting, your body adapts to it by consuming your body fat. It also has some psychological benefits as if you feel like you're not a slave to eating. Intermittent fasting is the best way to balance your fat loss and exercise routines. There is no better way than intermittent fasting to achieve maximum fat loss with a full workload.

Intermittent Fasting And Fat Loss

Intermittent fasting is a popular way to use your body's natural fat-burning ability to lose fat in a short amount of time. However, many people want to know if intermittent fasting works and how exactly it works. If you don't eat for a long time, your body changes the way it produces hormones and enzymes, which can have a positive effect on fat loss. These are the main benefits of fasting and how they achieve these benefits. Hormones are the basis for metabolic functions, such as the rate at which fat is burned. The growth hormone is developed in the body and promotes fat loss in the body to supply energy. If you fast for a while, your body begins to increase its growth hormone production. Fasting also reduces the amount of insulin in the blood, which ensures that your body burns fat instead of storing it. A short-term fast that lasts 12 to 72 hours increases your metabolism and adrenaline, which increases the number of calories burned. In addition, people who are fasting get more energy from more adrenaline, which means they don't feel tired, even though they generally don't get calories. Although you may think that fasting should reduce energy, the body balances it out and burns calories. Most people who eat every 3-5 hours burn sugar primarily, not fat. Prolonged fasting turns your metabolism into fat burning. At the end of a 24-hour fasting day, your body used up glycogen stores in the first few hours and spent approximately 18 of those hours burning the fat reserves in your body. For those who are regularly active but still struggling with fat loss, intermittent fasting can help increase fat loss without speeding up an exercise program or drastically changing a diet plan.

Another advantage of IF is that it essentially resets the human body. Spending a day or so without eating changes a person's desire and makes them feel less hungry over time. If you have difficulty eating consistently, intermittent fasting can help your body adjust to periods when you don't eat and help you not feel hungry all the time. Many people notice that if they temporarily fast one day a week, they start eating healthier and more controlled. Intermittent fasting varies but is generally advised for about a day a week. During this day, a person can have a liquid nutrient-filled smoothie or other low-calorie option. Since the body gets used to intermittent fasting, this is usually not necessary. Intermittent fasting helps to naturally reduce fat stores in the body by switching metabolism so that fat is broken down instead of sugar or muscle. It has been used effectively by many people and is an easy way to make a beneficial change. For anyone struggling with stubborn fat and fed up with the traditional diet, intermittent fasting offers a simple and effective option for fat loss and a healthier lifestyle.

Intermittent fasting has never been more popular in recent years! There are many celebrities, PTs, and influencers who praise fat loss! Many examine intermittent fasting to be a diet, but it is not. It's just a dietary pattern! This pattern includes cycling between mealtimes and non-meals. Eat only in certain time slots. And why is it becoming more and more popular? If the goal is fat loss, the theory behind intermittent fasting is that usually, you consume fewer calories during a set mealtime than if you were eating all day! Therefore, changing what you eat only when you eat is not a rule! That is why many people find this very simple and easy. It doesn't need a major change in behavior! This is most likely the reason that is so popular with many people. When do you fast and when to "feast"? There are many variations on intermittent fasting, but the most common is the 16-8 protocol. This involves 16 hours of fasting and 8 hours of meals daily. Again, at different times, most people eat between 12 pm and 8 pm. That would mean that they totally fast the 16 hours between 8 pm and 12 pm! The key is to choose a period that best fits your lifestyle, commitments, and schedule.

If your fitness goal is fat loss, you can think about intermittent fasting. If you eat for a limited period of time, you are more likely to have a calorie deficit, which will promote fat loss. It's a lot easier than dieting! You don't add new foods to your meals that you may not like; you simply change the pattern. If you choose intermittent fasting, check the different versions and find the one that suits you best! As with most things related to fitness, the best thing you can do is consistent and long-term! If you are currently eating every 1-2 hours, your desire will increase, at least in the short term. If you are always hungry, this strategy is probably not for you! Thinking is a big part of intermittent fasting. If you think about food all the time during Lent and it makes you unhappy or irritable, then it's probably not for you either.

The idea of fasting in a diet plan is often viewed very negatively in fitness culture. Many companies and trainers believe that if you don't eat every few hours, your metabolism will slow down, or our body will go into "hunger mode." Before we go any further, we have to realize that "slowing down metabolism" can be one of the biggest myths in the entire fitness industry. The metabolism has been reduced in recent weeks with chronic, low-calorie consumption. This is not the case if you fast several times a week. Here's a simple overview of how intermittent fasting is implemented in a person's schedule.

1. Eat normally until dinner (2-4 meals, not 6-8)

2. Eat your dinner, but stop eating afterward.

3. Fast until dinner the next day. (No calorie consumption)

4. For this meal, you just eat a normal dinner.

With this approach, you still fast for 24 hours, but eat something every day. This is usually done 1-2 times a week. If you want to lose a lot of weight before a vacation or reunion, you can fast three times a week.

What you learn about yourself while fasting

If you are fasting, be aware of any changes in the way you eat. If you've had a 24-hour fast a few times, you may be told the reasons for what, when, and why you eat. Many of the reasons why we eat are emotional connections or habits rather than actual hunger. Sometimes we are so conditioned at certain times that we eat a meal when we are not hungry.

When you say that like everything else it is the best option for you or not, it is important that you find out if it is and don't reject it until at least you've experimented with it. The benefits of intermittent fasting are amazing, and in combination with an appropriate exercise program and proper nutrition, you can build muscle according to bodybuilding standards. In certain circumstances, there is ample evidence that intermittent fasting can help burn fat. Intermittent fasting means that your last meal of the day and your first meal the next day are further up to 16 hours apart. This is because it takes your body about six to eight hours after eating to metabolize this glycogen and then getting it back into your fat stores to continue functioning. However, if we start feeding our bodies before this six to eight-year period or before using glycogen, we will never let our system access our fat stores. This makes it very difficult to lose weight. Of course, if you fast, you go too far.

When we exceed a certain point, our system recognizes that it is out of food and goes into hunger mode. At this point, it basically stops using our excess fat. Tests have shown that intermittent fasting has additional health benefits. These include increased insulin sensitivity, reducing oxidative stress, and increasing the ability to withstand cellular stress. All this delays the aging of the cells and prevents diseases that are associated with cell damage. So is an intermittent fasting plan suitable for everyone? In fact, all the factors that contribute to healthy weight loss make it almost impossible to find a magic ball that is right for everyone. First, it can be said with certainty that pregnant women should never fast. A baby needs all the nutrients it can get, and some studies have actually shown that fasting can change the baby's heartbeat and breathing patterns, along with increasing gestational diabetes. Those suffering from hypoglycemia, a condition with abnormally low blood sugar levels, should not go through periods of fasting. If you suffer from this disease, your goal is first to normalize your blood sugar level and then opt for a less rigid version of the fast. People with diabetes are also not helped with intermittent fasting.

Finally, you have to realize that if you drive too fast, you have to pay more attention to your diet while eating. If you continue on a toxic diet with highly processed foods and then don't eat for 15 or 16 hours, you can do more harm than good to your body in the long run. It is vital to put together a healthy eating plan to ensure that you get the right nutrition in the shorter time you eat. Whenever you make dramatic changes in your diet, even if they are healthy changes that ultimately benefit your health, it may take a while for your system to adapt to the change. But hear out what your body is saying to you, and if you're too fast, don't fight it. Just be a little slower with the changes, and if it is good for your system, it will adopt at some point.

A Common Question About Intermittent Fasts:

Are there any foods or drinks you can consume during intermittent fasting? Unless you're on the modified 5: 2 fasting diet (mentioned above), you shouldn't eat or drink anything that contains calories. Water, black coffee, and all foods/drinks that do not contain calories may be consumed during Lent. In fact, adequate water intake is essential during IF, and some say that drinking black coffee while fasting helps reduce hunger.

IF YOU WANT JUST THE BENEFITS:

Intermittent fasting research is still in its infancy, but still has great potential for weight loss and the treatment of some chronic diseases. To sum it up again, here are the possible benefits of intermittent fasting shown in Human Studies:

1. Weight loss

2. Improve fat blood markers like cholesterol

3. Reduce inflammation

4. Reduced stress and improved self-confidence

5. Improved mood

Shown in animal studies:

1. Reduced body fat

2. Decreased levels of the hunger hormone leptin

3. Improve insulin levels

4. Protect against obesity, fatty liver disease, and inflammation

5. Longevity

Before considering the benefits of intermittent fasting, understand why eating 5-6 meals a day or every few hours (the exact opposite of fasting) can actually do more harm than good. When we eat, we absorb food energy. The key hormone is insulin (produced by the pancreas), which increases during meals. Both carbohydrates and protein stimulate insulin. Fat triggers a lower insulin effect, but fat is rarely eaten alone. Insulin has two main functions - First, the body can immediately start using food energy. Carbohydrates are quickly converted to glucose, which increases blood sugar levels. Insulin directs glucose into the body's cells to use as energy. Protein is split into amino acids, and excess amino acids are converted to glucose. Protein does not necessarily increase blood sugar, but it can stimulate insulin. Fats have a minimal effect on insulin. Second, insulin stores excess energy for future use. Insulin converts excess glucose to glycogen and stores it in the liver. Despite that, there is a limit to the amount of glycogen that can be stored. As soon as the limit is reached, the liver begins to convert glucose to fat. Then, the fat is stored in the liver (which becomes excessive, fatty liver) or in fat deposits in the body (often stored as visceral or belly fat). Therefore, if we eat and eat all day, we are constantly fed, and the insulin level remains high. In other words, we may spend most of the day storing food.

What happens if you fast?

The process of using and storing dietary energy that occurs during a meal is reversed during a fast. The insulin level drops, and the body begins to burn stored energy. Glycogen, the glucose stored in the liver, is first retrieved and used. After that, the body begins to break down stored body fat for energy. Thus, the body basically exists in two states - the fed state with a high insulin level and the fasting state with a low insulin level. We either store food energy or burn food energy. When eating and fasting are balanced, there is no weight gain. If we spend most of the day eating and storing energy, there is a good chance that we will gain weight over time.

A Powerful Tool For Weight Loss And Diabetes: Intermittent Fasting

First of all, fasting is not hunger. Hunger is the involuntary abstinence from eating, which is forced by external forces. This happens in times of war and hunger when food is scarce. Fasting, on the other hand, is voluntary, intentional, and controlled. Food is readily available, but we choose not to eat it for spiritual, health, or other reasons. Fasting is as old as human beings and much older than any other trophic form. Ancient civilizations, like the Greeks, recognized that regular fasting was inherently beneficial. They have often been referred to as times of healing, cleansing, or detoxification. Virtually every culture and religion on earth practices some fasting rituals. Before the advent of agriculture, people never ate three meals a day and a snack in between. They only ate when they found a food that could be hours or days apart. From an evolutionary perspective, eating three meals a day is not a prerequisite for survival. Otherwise, they would not have survived as a species. Fasting has no standard duration. It can take anywhere from a few hours to many days to months. IF is an eating pattern in which we alternate between fasting and eating regularly. Shorter fasting periods of 16 to 20 hours are usually carried out even more frequently every day. Longer periods of fasting, usually 24 to 36 hours, are done 2-3 times a week. We all happen to fast for about 12 hours a day between dinner and breakfast. Fasting has been practiced by millions and millions of people for thousands of years. Is it unhealthy? In fact, numerous studies have shown that it has enormous health benefits.

The portion control strategy of constant calorie reduction is the most common nutritional recommendation for weight loss and type 2 diabetes. Intermittent fasting is not a constant calorie restriction. Limiting calories leads to a compensatory increase in hunger and, worse, a decrease in the body's metabolism, a double curse! Because if we burn fewer calories a day, it becomes increasingly difficult to lose weight, and it is much easier to regain weight after losing it. This type of diet puts the body in a "hunger mode" because the metabolism works to save energy.

Intermittent weight loss during fasting is one of the most effective ways to lose extra pounds. The ideas of intermittent fasting for weight loss call into question most of the beliefs held so far about losing. Those looking for new approaches to lose weight effectively accepted their ideas immediately. You are probably tired of trying something with the word "diet" when it comes to weight loss. IF is a way of eating that includes a structured program of eating and not eating, if the program can be processed, build the program all day if desired. If you continue the program, you can extend your Lent later. Of course, you know the more weight you eat and the more weight you want and eat. If you are using an intermittent program, you may need to eat less frequently. Sometimes you have to do without breakfast.

May sleep for 6-8 hours. During this time, your body is in hungry mode. When your body is fasting, it usually produces more insulin. As insulin in the body increases, insulin sensitivity in the body increases. If your body has increased insulin sensitivity, you lose more fat. If your body has increased insulin sensitivity, you will lose more fat. The brilliance of the intermittent fasting weight loss program is that you skip breakfast to increase your body's insulin sensitivity. This means your body will be in fat reduction mode for a long time. You will lose more weight. A longer fasting mode also works well for growth hormone levels in your body. If you skip breakfast or eat for a period of time, your body produces growth hormone. The growth hormone is what your body is supposed to produce when you are trying to lose weight. This is simply because the growth hormone promotes weight loss in your body. Growth hormone levels typically peak when using an intermittent fasting weight loss program. During this time, you lose weight. Upper levels of growth hormone in the body have several other health benefits. This program is incredible!

Intermittent fasting weight loss programs are fundamentally different from most weight loss programs advertised on the market. How do you want: better control over your hunger, an easy way to lose fat and build lean, attractive muscles, increased insulin sensitivity, reduced inflammation, increased growth hormone, a super-efficient method of eliminating toxins, the freedom to eat everything you want without guilt? We were all told that you have to train consistently and with a lot of intensity to lose weight. Regular training is important to maintain health and burn fat, but the question arises: "Is exercise really enough? No. Without changing your diet, it is practically impossible to lose weight and keep it off consistently. Here, most people avoid diet and exercise because conventional wisdom states that you have to deprive yourself of the foods you enjoy to lose weight. Intermittent weight loss during fasting is not necessarily a new concept. In many cultures, fasting is an integral part of life for both cultural and religious reasons. In these cases, fasting is not done to reduce weight, but to cleanse the body. In place of fasting for days or weeks, the IF practitioner (intermittent fasting) fasts between 16 and 20 hours a day. A typical day most people eat is something like this:

8:00 am breakfast

12:00 noon lunch

7:00 pm dinner

Maybe a light snack before bed. This schedule means that the meal is spread over a mealtime of 12 hours or more. Intermittent fasting allows you to eat relatively equal amounts of food within a compressed time frame. An intermittent weight loss plan for fasting would look something like this:

10:00 am breakfast

2 pm lunch

6 pm dinner

What we did effectively is to compress the dining window to 8 hours. Only water should be consumed outside the 8-hour window. This has several major advantages. Eat less, to begin with, as most people don't usually digest their food quickly enough to eat the same amount of food that they would consume in a larger dining window. Eating less food while making the same amount of effort every day means weight loss. As more water is consumed, your body also has more options for flushing out excess sodium and waste material. There is a mental adjustment period of approximately 2 weeks. This is the time it usually takes your body and mind to get used to the changes in eating. After two weeks, hunger subsides. Intermittent fasting benefits the practitioner in several ways.

Several studies and experiments have been conducted over the years to determine the effectiveness of weight loss through intermittent fasting. The term intermittent fasting basically means dividing the day into zones; there will be eating zones, and others will be fasting zones. Popularly known as eating windows and fasting, the key is to maintain proportions while working in the gaps. Weight loss through this medium is easier than intensive training or especially nursing mothers who cannot afford the time to go to a gym or workout. Intermittent fasting is exactly what people want to do, eat whatever they want, namely chocolates, cream, and other fat products, and let the calories go into deficit. To get an overview of intermittent fasting and how weight loss with its convention occurs in daily lifestyle, here is a brief summary of how to practice and benefit from it.

1) Select the 24-hour IF technique or the 12-hour window. There are several types of intermittent fasting plans that can be set. Some vary from 24 hours plus, which means that you eat on Tuesday at 6 pm and then take your next meal on Wednesday at 6 pm fasting as long as this should not be encouraged as such because it affects the metabolic rate and, in turn, deteriorates health. The better option is to choose a 12-hour window in which to fast half a day and then all the beneficial fat or carbohydrate foods. What happens is when a meal is ingested, the body uses it for the next 12 hours, and when it is digested, the calories that are stored as fat are burned and used by the body. This causes weight loss, and after a while, the urge and starvation attacks disappear when the body gets used to it.

2) Keep the diet simple and short. Weight loss through intermittent fasting

only occurs if it is practiced consistently. For consistency, there should be a plan that is simple and easy to follow on a daily basis. Fix groups of food at 12-hour intervals and have only these. Simply balancing the groups would determine the food intake that is essential for the well-being of the body, the good metabolism, and finally, the burning out of weight in an unexpected way. The group can contain calcium, fiber, carbohydrates, and fats. The only thing is to balance it appropriately.

3) Reduces the strain on the body, which has to eat something again and again. Intermittent fasting basically shapes the body's needs so that the need for frequent snacking automatically subsides. So what happens is the time when extra food and fat that is used to store in the body simply removes that particular time from the daily routine and weight loss begins. The stress that the body incurred when processing, digesting, and using the fat and the additional meal is also reduced. Instead, the same amount of energy is used to digest the stored calories and burned by reducing fat in the stomach and in other parts of the body.

4) Blood sugar levels and routines are adjusted accordingly. Intermittent fasting has several health benefits, and one of them is a balanced blood sugar level as your body's intake decreases. Studies show that fewer cravings occur, and, in addition to the sugar level, blood pressure, stress, and heart diseases are brought under control by this form of the diet. This would not only avoid strict workouts and not make hard food cuts, but it would also eat almost anything you could wish for in a few months while still reducing weight. In addition, there is healthier and more nutritious food intake over time, and it is difficult to get used to if IF is not followed.

Losing weight is not that difficult. In fact, it is very simple. This may sound impossible to most people, and they may think this is a lie, but in fact, it is not. Losing a few pounds while building muscle in a few weeks is not a dream. How? It's not the complicated overeating. It is not an expensive, rare, and nutritious supplement or food. It is not the program to eat small meals six times a day. It is not one of these programs that does not promise much for a live program. Don't be surprised, but the answer is intermittent fasting. This may sound ridiculous to some, but this is not a joke for research. Short-term fasting or intermittent fasting research has shown what a great program it is, and when you consider that it is not the same with diets. Flexible intermittent fasting means you don't have to starve or drool like crazy when you take a look at delicious food. It is adaptable and does not prevent you from eating your favorite food. The research carried out has shown that this so-called fasting increases the burning enzyme in the body, which is why people lose weight much more easily if they do not work harder. That is the purpose of this program. It is the simplest and fastest way to lose weight. Stop working so hard with weight loss programs that don't give you the result you should get. Do not worry about energy during intermittent fasting. Many people who fasted at short notice prove that they feel energized and most productive when fasting. This is because fasting does not affect your metabolism. Shape your body and maintain your health with what works because you cannot buy health and beauty unless you take action.

Intermittent Fasting Bodybuilding For Increase Energy

It's no secret that intermittent fasting helps rejuvenate a person's body and fitness. During intermittent fasting, the person only consumes water, juices, or other low-calorie substances. It means a time of eating, followed by a time of not eating. However, water alone during fasting helps cleanse the body and drive out the contaminants in the body. In many cultures, intermittent fasting in China is more or less mandatory for everyone, which enables people from these parts of the world to be very agile and fit. Fasting and bodybuilding are often linked. To build the body, it is extremely important that the body is fit. Intermittent fasting is one of the most natural or effective methods to keep the body fit, as it helps by expelling the body's impurities and giving the various organs involved in digesting food their quota of much-needed rest. Therefore, the person will feel more comfortable and happy with themselves. This in-depth feeling of well-being increases trust in the person and motivates them to build up the body. Intermittent fasting bodybuilding is, therefore, a natural way to improve fitness levels.

For beginners, the concept of intermittent bodybuilding fasting seems to be a Herculean task and can easily give up in a short amount of time, but it must be understood that fasting helps itself at regular intervals and its self-confidence over a period of time. Perseverance must be maintained in order to achieve the best results. There is another tendency that we should be very careful about, and it is not about going overboard and stressing yourself. Usually, people are in a hurry to get fit and build the body of their dreams quickly too much to get sick; it should be avoided. This can be avoided by paying attention to the various pointers and tips that the body gives you. As if you were eating something when you feel very dizzy or a little too tired, or other symbols the body sends to indicate that it desperately needs calories. There is no reason for fasting for a while and then in calories immediately after you stop fasting. Instead, slowly take in calories and exercise the way you want to, so as not to injure yourself or overdo the exercises. Fasting and bodybuilding are one of the oldest and most proven methods to cleanse your body and keep it in good shape. This helps you to keep your body in shape and gives you the much-needed trust in yourself. Above all, you recognize the value of food and its importance. Similarly, it also creates one of the basic building blocks for bodybuilding, as it is essential to building a body that has a conditioned body. If your body is not in the right condition, you must get it right the old way with intermittent fasting. Better control of hunger, an easy way to lose fat, build lean and attractive muscle, increase insulin sensitivity, reduce inflammation, increase growth hormone, and a very efficient way to remove toxins.

In a traditional fat loss routine, you want to cause a calorie deficit. It doesn't matter how you cause this deficit. All that matters is that it is created. You can do this by diet or exercise alone, or you can combine the two. Preferably using a combination of the two is the best route. Since we have compared the two, we will keep them separately. When you exercise, the level of insulin in your blood drops. You will also see that hormone levels of human growth hormone (HGH) increase when you exercise intensely. These conditions are necessary for fat loss to take place. It has been studied, and it has been shown that fasting for only 24 hours can produce the same hormone blood levels that are achieved by exercise. So if you just fasted once or twice a week for about 24 hours, you can reproduce the effects of the exercise without having to exercise at all. This is good news for those who hate exercising or just don't have enough time to exercise.

What to Expect From Intermittent Fasting?

The hunger is going down - We usually feel hungry about four hours after eating. So if we fast 24 hours, does that mean that our hunger feelings are six times as strong? Of course not. Many people fear that fasting will lead to extreme hunger and overeating. Studies have shown that the day after a one-day fast, calorie intake actually increases by 20%. With repeated fasting, however, hunger and appetite surprisingly decrease. Hunger comes in waves. If we do nothing, the hunger will disappear after a while. Drinking tea (of all kinds) or coffee (with or without caffeine) is often enough to ward off it. However, one or two teaspoons of cream will not cause much insulin response, but it is best to drink in black. Do not use sugar or artificial sweeteners at all. Bone soup can be consumed during fasting if needed.

Blood sugar doesn't crash - Sometimes, people fear that during fasting, the blood sugar will become very low, and they will be shaky and sweaty. This doesn't really happen because the body closely monitors the blood sugar, and there are several mechanisms to keep it in the right area. During fasting, the body breaks down glycogen in the liver and begins to release glucose. This happens every night during sleep. If we fast for more than 24 to 36 hours, the glycogen stores are used up, and the liver produces new glucose using glycerin, which is a by-product of fat loss (a process called gluconeogenesis). In addition to using glucose, our brain cells can also use ketones for energy. Ketones are created when fat is metabolized and can meet up to 75% of the brain's energy requirements (the other 25% from glucose). The only exception is for those who take diabetes and insulin. You MUST consult your doctor first as the dosages will likely need to be reduced during fasting. Otherwise, if you overdose the drug and experience dangerous hypoglycemia, you need sugar to reverse it. This breaks fast and is counterproductive.

The phenomenon of dawn - After fasting, especially in the morning, some people suffer from high blood sugar. This dawn phenomenon is the result of the daily rhythm in which the body releases higher levels of hormones shortly before waking up to prepare for the day ahead.

Adrenaline-gives energy to the body

Growth hormone-repair and production of new proteins

Glucagon-Glucose is transported from the liver reservoir to the blood for use as energy

Cortisol, stress hormone-activates the body

These hormones peak in the morning and then fall to low levels during the day. In non-diabetics, the level of blood sugar increase is small, and most people will not even notice it. In the majority of diabetics, however, there can be a noticeable increase in blood sugar levels if the liver pours sugar into the blood. This will also happen in extended fasts. When there is no food, the insulin level remains low while the liver releases some of its stored sugar and fat. This is natural and not a bad thing at all. The size of the tip decreases when the liver is less inflated with sugar and fat.

IF is a feeding pattern that alternates between periods of fasting and dietary restrictions, it is a simple diet method that is divided into many types. One of the intermittent fasting methods is fasting on the second day, in which a person takes a normal diet on certain days of the week and fasts on some. During the fasting days, one does not completely do without food but reduces the calorie intake to 1/4 of the normal diet. The other type of fasting is that eating within a day is limited to a certain time window. This means that eating is restricted to 8 hours of eating by the window, which means that one person eats once every eight hours. However, some people reduce the time to six, four, or even two hours as needed. The longest time a person can stay on intermittent fasting without food is 36 hours. When used appropriately, this can lead to a number of positive health effects. For example, intermittent fasting promotes general health. It significantly reduces the craving for snacks and sugar. Practice normalizes both insulin and leptin sensitivity. Insulin resistance contributes to many chronic diseases, such as diabetes, cancer, and heart infections. Intermittent fasting, therefore, protects the body against such infections. Intermittent fasting improves brain health. Fasting helps the body convert stored glycogen to glucose to release energy. If fasting continues for some time, the continued breakdown of body fat will cause the liver to secrete ketone bodies. These small molecules are by-products of fatty acid synthesis and can be used as fuel by the brain. Research also shows that exercise and fasting lead to genes and other growth factors that are essential for the recycling and rejuvenation of the brain.

This type of fasting also promotes physical fitness and weight loss. Combined fasting and training increases the effects of catalysts and cellular factors so that the breakdown of glycogen and fats is maximized. When you exercise hungry, the body is forced to burn stored fats for significant weight loss. The program is also known to prevent cognitive decline. In 2006, studies were conducted on mice using water labyrinth tests to assess the cognitive functions of mice with a normal diet and with intermittent fasting. It was discovered that mice that fasted intermittently experienced slower cognitive decline, which also applies to humans. Intermittent fasting also promotes muscle building, especially in men. This is because after eating, the energy gained is used to maintain a workout. However, if the workout is done during fasting, the body uses stored body fats to maintain the exercises. Eating after the session ensures that the energy gained is used to replenish the body optimally. This helps the muscles to recover and build up quickly. In summary, intermittent fasting is a healthy practice, but it can lead to depression in people who cannot fully maintain it. It takes commitment and perseverance to manage the change in diet, as only consistency can achieve these positive results.

How do you want: better control over your hunger, an easy way to lose fat and build lean, attractive muscles, increased insulin sensitivity, reduced inflammation, increased growth hormone, a super-efficient method of eliminating toxins, the freedom to eat everything you want without guilt? The diet that you follow during intermittent fasting depends on the results you are looking for, and you are assuming. If you want to lose a major amount of weight, you need to scrutinize your diet, but if you want to lose a few pounds on the beach, you may be able to do so by continuing intermittent fasting for several weeks. There are several ways to make a fast. The basic method is to fast 24 hours twice a week. It makes sense to do this every few days. It's easier to choose a day that you're busy, so you don't get distracted by hunger. You may have hunger pangs at first, but they go away, and once you get used to intermittent fasting, you may find that you feel that hunger poses no problem for you anymore. You may find that when you fast, you have a lot of focus and focus, which is contrary to what you would expect, but many people experience this.

Advantageous Low-Carb Intermittent Fasting

Low carb diets can mean limiting carbohydrates to 100 or even 50 grams a day. This means reducing sugar, starch, and all carbohydrate foods. Of course, this is better for your body because your pancreas doesn't have to work as hard to remove sugar from your system. Intermittent fasting means fasting for a certain period of time. This means that your body has to search for food (fuel), thereby removing badly aged or damaged cells and other waste that has accumulated in your body. Combine the two for "Low Carb Intermittent Fasting," and you have a winning combination to lose weight and feel great! If you're fasting, you can still have low-carb and low-calorie drinks like water and black coffee, but you shouldn't eat food for 24 hours. You can eat a healthy diet the next day, but you should still keep an eye on your carbohydrate intake. Read labels and research for food to know you're making the best decisions for your body and health. "Live" or fresh food, is always a good choice. Remember, junk-in means junk-out, and healthy choices mean a healthier lifestyle. This is a lifestyle change and should be a consistent way of eating for you (at least the low carbohydrates). You have to work diligently to make a smart choice of food and drink! Combine intermittent low-carb fasting with exercise, and you'll be in shape before you know it and feel fantastic. Intermittent fasting reduces fat oxidation and can reduce body weight. Training speeds up the process and helps you get rid of sagging skin and tighten yourself.

Intermittent fasting performed on animals shows an increase in lifespan by 40% or more. That is amazing! This shows how much healthy eating and cleansing your body can not only benefit your system and help you lose weight, but can also extend your days on earth. Low carb food choices are vegetables. You can eat as many vegetables as you like. Meat and fish are a good choice for dinner. For lunch, you can make a salad with a boiled egg, onions, and a hint of cheese. Watch the carbohydrates in the dressing. As long as you are determined to choose a healthy lifestyle, your desire for sugar and carbohydrates will most likely have disappeared. This wish will definitely be reduced! You no longer want fatty, sweet foods if you choose healthy, low-carb foods. Drink lots of water too. Other drinks that are good are black coffee and green tea but don't overdo the caffeine. And remember, before you start on a diet plan or exercise routine, always consult your doctor! You want to make sure you stay healthy while becoming healthier!

Adjust and reduce the amount of time you get to eat than the number of calories you ingest. Aside from losing weight, it also has many health benefits

• It reduces your urge to get hungry during a diet. Controlling this hunger is definitely a daunting task for someone who wants to start a diet. But after a few days of starting intermittent fasting, your body adapts to this new eating behavior.

• It increases your mental focus and concentration. As you indulge in fasting, your body releases the chemical called catecholamines, which significantly increases your mental awareness and productivity.

• It stabilizes your energy level and improves your mood. Your blood sugar level remains stable with fewer meals. This leads to a constant energy level and helps you to avoid diabetes in the long term.

• Reduced oxidative stress. This simply means that the build-up of oxidative radicals in the body is reduced during fasting. This significantly reduces damage to internal orgasms in your body.

• It increases your ability to withstand stress, disease, and aging. Intermittent fasting, like exercise, induces a cellular stress response in your body that increases your ability to deal with stress and resist disease and aging.

• You can burn fat. Obviously, this is the main reason. You can lose excess weight. When you eat, your body uses the glycogen from the food you just ate to give you energy. But when you fast, your body switches to the stored fats and uses them for energy.

• You save time and money. Eating fewer meals means preparing and buying fewer meals. This saves you money and time. Plus, you're less exposed to flavors, so you're less bored and eat something you shouldn't.

You may have heard of calorie restrictions to extend our lives, but did you know that there is a healthier alternative in the form of intermittent fasting? Intermittent fasting is a great way to continue gaining weight with the Paleo diet after an initial weight loss. Intermittent fasting (IF) increases your fat metabolism. As long as you keep your fast at a reasonable limit, for example, 24 to 36 hours, your metabolism will speed up, and more fat cells will be burned than you have trained with the Paleo diet. Intermittent fasting does not reduce your muscle mass like a calorie restriction. Calorie reduction has a more harmful effect on your skeletal muscle than intermittent fasting. Intermittent fasting helps remove waste. Autophagy is a process in which waste material is removed from your cells, and this process is initiated by fasting. Often people tend to use IF once a week because of problems with work, school, and social eating with others. Though, you can do this up to three times a week or daily in smaller sessions. It is best if each person decides what works for their body by trying it out. The key is to start slowly, so you don't realize early that it's too difficult to deal with. One method is to have breakfast one day and then not have breakfast until the next day or choose another meal to do so as you like. Not to mention that IF offers other benefits as well. Some of these benefits include protection against Alzheimer's through increased production of BDNF (neurotropic factor from the brain), lowering cholesterol and triglycerides, increased insulin sensitivity, and a longer lifespan. Other more anecdotal benefits include mental clarity and greater resistance to stress. An interesting side effect for those paleo dieters interested in weight lifting and exercise is that intermittent fasting can increase growth hormone, especially in men. The growth hormone has many benefits for adults, including increased muscle mass and skin effects that help create a youthful look. Also, don't worry that this will affect your workout. Studies of athletes who have exercised during fasting have shown that this has little or no effect on their performance. In some cases, it can improve athletes' metabolic balance to reduce body fat rather than muscle better.

The Role Of Hormones

Hormones play a crucial role in our bodies. Every hormone has its function and performance. Our growth hormone helps us burn fat. When we fast, our growth hormone starts working overtime and burning fat much faster. Fasting also keeps our insulin levels low, so we burn the fat instead of storing it in our body. In order for our hormones to burn fat, they also need fat-burning enzymes. Fat tissue HSL and muscle tissue LPL are the two most important fat-burning enzymes. HSL helps the body release fat and convert it into energy and muscles, while LPL helps the cells in our muscles to store the fat so that it can be burned as fuel. When these enzymes work together, they help hormones burn fat twice as fast. By intermittent fasting, these hormones and enzymes can quickly burn the fat on the day you fast.

Fasting is a great way to keep your body and mind healthy and clean. Many people who fast intermittently claim that they have learned a lot about their eating habits. The reason is that they have plenty of time to think about food and what foods they crave on their fasting days. The level of adrenaline your body produces is also increased during short-term fasting, which makes your body's ability to burn fat faster and work twice as hard. Combine this with your increased metabolism, and you can see how often losing weight with intermittent fasting would be.

WHO SHOULD NOT DO INTERMITTENT FASTING?

Women who want to become pregnant or pregnant or breastfeeding. Contraindications Avoid intermittent fasting if you are pregnant, diabetic, have a serious illness, or are taking prescribed medication. If in doubt, it is leading to contact your doctor.

Those who are malnourished or underweight. Children under the age of 18 and the elderly. Those who have gout. Those who have gastroesophageal reflux disease (GERD). People with eating disorders should consult their doctor first. Those taking diabetic medication and insulin need to consult their doctor first because the dosage needs to be reduced.

Those taking medication should consult their doctor first, as the timing of medication can be affected. Those who feel very stressed or who have cortisol problems should not fast because fasting is another stress factor. Those who train very hard most days of the week should not fast

How Do You Prepare For Intermittent Fasting?

If someone is thinking about starting intermittent fasting, it is best to switch to a low-carb, high-fat diet for three weeks first. This allows the body to get used to using fat instead of glucose as an energy source. This means that all sugar, grains (bread, cookies, pastries, pasta, rice), legumes, and refined vegetable oils are removed. This minimizes most of the side effects associated with fasting. Start with a shorter fast of 16 hours, for example, from dinner (8 pm) to lunch (12 pm) the next day. You can usually eat between 12 noon and 8 p.m., and you can eat either two or three meals. As soon as you feel comfortable with it, you can extend the fast to 18, 20 hours. For shorter fasts, you can do it continuously every day. For longer fasts, such as 24-36 hours, you can do it 1-3 times a week, alternating between fasting and normal eating days. There is no real fasting program. The key is to choose one that works best for you. Some people get results with shorter fasts; others may need longer fasts. Some people do classic fasting only with water, others quickly make tea and coffee, and others quickly make a broth. No matter what you do, it is very important to stay hydrated and monitor yourself. If at any time you feel sick, you should stop immediately. You can be hungry, but you shouldn't feel sick.

INTERMITTENT FASTING FOR BEGINNERS

Intermittent fasting for beginners has two rules: (1) Fasting must be pleasant and NOT stressful. (2) Fasting must be simple and NOT rigid. There are two main reasons for people who want to do intermittent fasting - weight loss or health, or both. In any case, it is good to keep these two formulas in mind:

More rules = more complicated = little chance of success

Fewer rules = less complicated = high chances of success

In terms of health, a 24-hour break is very healthy, it helps you reduce calories without sacrificing what you like to eat on days without fasting, and perhaps more importantly, it stimulates your body to produce more growth hormone. Yes, that's the right growth hormone, the same thing you hear about the celebrities who strive to stay young. The growth hormone has many anti-aging benefits, and one of the most interesting is fat burning! In an ideal situation, 2 sessions of 24-hour fasting per week are good enough to achieve significant health and weight loss benefits. However, beginners are not advised to start fasting 24 hours unless you are absolutely sure that you can do so. There is no standard rule for IF. Just try it out and let it work for you. Let simplicity and flexibility be your fasting motto. Don't make yourself stressed. As a beginner to intermittent fasting, "Get rid of other weight loss methods and focus on IF." This is your first step to IF success. Think about how many times you've been told that breakfast is the most important meal in a day, or you need to eat 6 to 10 small meals a day to lose weight. We are not saying that these rules are wrong. If these rules work for you, stick to them. However, if you are on the path of intermittent fasting, you should better put these concepts aside for at least the time you are trying IF. Do you have your IF mindset ready? Then start with "skip meal" and see how your body reacts. Select a day to skip breakfast. Instead, drink fresh juice, water, or tea. No coffee, please. If that works well, try skipping lunch and proceed gradually. Anyone can do a 24 hour fast with an appropriate fasting setting. A useful tip is not to think about food. Avoid social talks in the pantry during lunch. Go for a walk or do some simple exercises. You can also examine these IF options:

• Shortened dining window, e.g., Eat ONLY between 11 am and 5 pm;

• Skip the meal unscheduled as far as it is natural and does not affect your daily work.

• Early and late, i.e., skip lunch;

• One meal a day, ideally only when you are relaxed and really have time to enjoy your meal.

To repeat it, fasting must be pleasant and not stressful. Do not press hard on yourself. Be flexible. It is very important. Do not upset your boss when you are invited to a business lunch by telling him that you are fasting. Do as you see fit, and your schedule allows.

Intermittent Fasting For Women

For women interested in weight loss, intermittent fasting may seem like a good choice, but many people want to know if women should fast. Is intermittent fasting effective in women? There are some important intermittent fasting studies that can help shed light on this interesting new nutritional trend. Intermittent fasting is also known as fasting on the second day, although there are certainly some variations on this diet. On the fasting days, the participants consumed food at 25% of their estimated energy requirements. The rest of the time, they received nutritional advice. Intermittent fasting in women has some positive effects. What makes it particularly important for women trying to lose weight is that women have a much higher percentage of fat in their bodies. When trying to lose weight, the body burns primarily from carbohydrate stores for the first 6 hours and then begins to burn fat. Women who eat healthily and exercise may have stubborn fat problems, but fasting is a realistic solution.

Obviously, our bodies and metabolism change when we go through menopause. One of the biggest changes women over 50 experience is that they have a slower metabolism and start to gain weight. However, fasting can be a great way to reverse and prevent weight gain. Studies have shown that this fasting pattern helps regulate appetite and that people who follow it regularly don't have the same cravings as others. If you are over 50 and are trying to adapt to your slower metabolism, intermittent fasting can help you avoid overeating. When you are 50 years old, your body also begins to develop some chronic diseases such as high cholesterol and high blood pressure. Intermittent fasting has been shown to lower both cholesterol and blood pressure, even without major weight loss. If you find that your numbers increase in the doctor's office every year, you may be able to lower them by fasting without losing much weight. Intermittent fasting may not be a good idea for every woman. Anyone with a certain health condition or who is hypoglycemic should consult a doctor. However, this new nutritional trend has specific advantages for women who naturally store more fat in their bodies and who may have problems getting rid of these fat reserves.

HOW TO SELECT THE BEST INTERMITTENT FASTING REGIME FOR YOU

Intermittent fasting improves health, reduces the risk of serious illness, and promotes longevity. You may be intrigued and want to try it out, but I don't know how to get started. Or maybe you experienced it once or twice and found it too difficult. There are three main methods for intermittent fasting: a) eat only from 6 p.m. to bedtime each day, b) fast around the clock on changing days, or c) one or two 36-hour fasts a week. It is worth experimenting with all three strategies to find out which ones are best for you in terms of your lifestyle and how they affect your health and well-being. Choose a day that is not too hectic or strenuous as it can lead to detoxification reactions. Make sure you have the opportunity to relax if necessary. You will get more out of the experience if you take the time to turn inward, calm the mind, meditate, think, and listen to your inner guidance. Ask for help from people near you before you start. It is great to fast with your partner so that you can motivate each other and share experiences. Eat the night lightly before by choosing a large salad or steamed vegetables with some lean protein. It makes no sense to eat the night before because it makes you feel hungrier while you are fasting. It's also best to avoid alcohol. Keep hydrated while fasting as your body has a significant need for fluids. Water, herbal teas, and vegetable juices are good choices. Drink at least 2 liters of liquid during the day. Avoid coffee, tea, carbonated drinks, fruit juices, and alcohol. Take 1 or 2 glasses of vegetable juice as it provides important electrolytes and has a health-promoting alkalizing effect. Try juicing celery, cucumber, chicory, fennel, and watercress. Avoid carrots and beets as they contain a lot of sugar.

Don't fight hunger because you will most likely do it. Just be senseless without judgment instead of opposing it. Take part in light exercises such as walking, stretching, and gentle yoga. This is not the day for an intense workout in the gym or something too vigorous. Add some breathing exercises like yogic pranayama. A few minutes of exercise offer amazing benefits from detoxification to increasing energy. Expect some detoxification symptoms like headache, drowsiness, or short periods of time when you feel nervous. These are made worse if you normally have a lot of caffeine and sugar in your diet. Avoid taking over-the-counter medications to reduce these side effects. Instead, rest, go for a walk and practice breathing exercises. Listen to your body wisdom and if you feel uncomfortable or it gets too much, take something to eat. Your body knows best. Carefully break the fast the next morning. Drink water or herbal tea and a piece of fruit when you get up and have breakfast as usual 30 minutes later. Eat the rest of the day as usual (you probably won't feel the need to overeat).

Enjoy the changes in your feelings during and after fasting. Notice changes in your energy, emotions, and mental state. You may find that eating the day after fasting is far more pleasant because your senses are sharpened. Recognize that it can take a few tries to get used to this practice. After a few weeks, your body will get used to it, and the benefits you will feel will increase as the symptoms decrease.

Everyone always wonders what's the next big secret in the diet industry ... In particular, people want to burn fat and build muscle while trying as little as possible. They want everything, and sometimes that takes a little too much. At least with most programs.

Breakfast is the major meal of the day:

This myth is easy to kill. Those who fast regularly (often from sleep to lunch, which means that breakfast is skipped) report an increased focus, an increased energy level, and a better mood when fasting. Are you looking for your new coffee? You have found one that burns fat and gives you energy.

Eating 6 meals a day speeds up your metabolism:

If you consume the identical number of calories and have the same macronutrient distribution (mostly via protein), eating those calories and nutrients makes 6 meals and 1 almost 0 difference. Because in the final analysis, if you use both methods to reduce calories, there is the same calorie deficit, and if you add calories, there is the same excess! And if there was a difference, you tend to think it is for the fasting method. By increasing insulin sensitivity, intermittent fasting can ensure that the calories get directly into your muscles when you eat! And if you are not fasting, the increased adrenaline/noradrenaline gives you energy and burns fat!

How To Organize An Intermittent Fasting Diet?

Here is the most basic summary of how it works:

* Eat 9 hours a day on training days and fast for the remaining 15 hours.

* Eat 6 hours a day on free or cardio days and fast for the remaining 18 hours.

* Strength training 3 days a week

* Cardio 2-4 times a week

* Maintain diet on weight training days + 500 calories

* Eat 50% of maintenance on other days. This plan is also inherent in fat loss.

Skip Meals - This can be done on a planned or unplanned basis. The key is not to make up for the missed meal with more food than you would normally eat at your next meal.

Shortening the meal window - This means that you take your first meal later in the day and your last meal earlier than normal. This quickly leads to longer night time.

Two meals - one meal at the beginning of the day and one at the end of the day.

Fasting every other day - This is very aggressive fasting and should only be done for a week and only once or twice a year.

Fasting 24 Hours - This is the most common method of fasting and losing weight. It is usually done from dinner one evening to dinner the next evening and once or twice a week.

With all fasting, it is important to resist the temptation to eat more at the next meal or the next time without fasting. You will want to eat more psychologically, but it won't be necessary as long as you keep eating healthy. By consuming more calories compared with the one your body can consume, you are increasing your reduced fat accumulation on an empty stomach.

Set eating/fasting times - The time of day you eat depends on whether you lift weights that day or not. Your meal window is 9 hours on lifting days and 6 hours on or off days. You need to be able to exercise weight and do cardio at the same time of day, as this disrupts the schedule.

After you've set your eating/fasting schedule, it's time to find out how many calories, fat, carbohydrates, and protein you're going to eat. This may seem overwhelming with all of the math, but once you've set your requirements, it's really quite simple and routine.

To find out the calories needed to lose fat, you first need to identify the calories required for maintenance. The simplest method to get an estimate is to multiply your weight by 15 in pounds. For instance, if you weigh 200 pounds, the total calories required for maintenance is 3000 calories per day.

Calorie requirements for strength training days: To determine calories on strength training days, take the number of maintenance calories, and add 500. To determine calorie consumption for off or cardio days, simply split your maintenance calories in half. For off or cardio days, our 200-pound person would eat 1500 calories a day. After your calorie needs for fat loss have been determined, it's time to find out how much of each macronutrient you need. The amounts vary depending on whether you do weight training that day or not. The macronutrients that we're going to use are the big three:

* Fat

* Protein

* Carbohydrates

(Note that fat is 9 calories per gram and protein and carbohydrates are 4 calories per gram)

Fat: The maximum fat intake per day is 30 grams. As long as ten of these grams are in the form of omega-3 fish oil, the origin of the fat is irrelevant.

Protein: To find out the minimum amount of protein per day, multiply your body weight by 1.25. Our 200 lb person needs at least 250 g of protein to maintain muscle. Sources don't matter, but be careful not to exceed the fat limit. Chicken, very lean red meat, non-fat cheese, and protein powder (whey or casein) are best.

Carbohydrates: Carbohydrates concoct the remaining calories in the diet. Again, the source is irrelevant. Here, too, the sources are irrelevant. Just be careful not to exceed the 30g fat limit and keep the sugar below 100g. In our example, he gets 270 calories from fat and 1000 calories from protein. With a calorie goal of 3500 lifting days, 2230 calories remain for carbohydrates. Divide 2230 by 4, and you get a maximum amount of carbohydrates of ~ 558 grams.

Macronutrient breakdown for days without lifting or cardio:

The calories needed for days when you don't exercise or do cardio are half of your maintenance calories. Here is the breakdown of macronutrients:

Fat: Again, the amount of fat remains unchanged compared to the training day. The maximum fat intake per day is 30 grams. As long as ten of these grams are in the form of omega-3 fish oil, the origin of the fat is irrelevant.

Carbohydrates: On rest days or aerobic exercise days, the carbohydrate source must be derived solely from fibrous green vegetables and trace components found in protein sources such as whey and cheese. The maximum amount per day should not surpass 20 grams.

Protein: The minimum amount of protein is pounds x 1.25 units of body weight. For subjects who need 1500 calories a day, she gets 80 calories from carbohydrates, 270 calories from fat, and the remaining 1150 calories from protein. This equates to about 287.5 grams.

Diet For Strength Training Days

Weight training will be 3 days a week, a whole-body routine. Use Monday-Wednesday-Friday, but the days are yours as long as there is a day off between training sessions. On training days, fasting is broken with a whey protein/carbohydrate shake 15 to 30 minutes before training begins.

Protein = 0.25 g / lb x weight Carbohydrates = 0.25 g / lb x weight

Gatorade powder or a maltodextrin/dextrose mixture is a preferred carbohydrate before training. Keep the fat to a minimum.

After training

You have another shake within 30 minutes of training. However, this time uses a mixture of whey, casein, and dextrose.

Protein = 0.25 g / lb x weight Carbohydrates = 0.50 g / lb x weight

The rest of the day

The first solid meal of the day is one hour after the PWO shake. This will be the major meal of the day. The remaining mealtimes are up to you, but reduce your calories until your last meal. Remember that with intermittent fasting, you don't have to eat every 2-3 hours. Just make sure you reach your calorie/macronutrient goals. However, casein shakes just before mealtime. Since it is a slowly digestible protein, it helps you stay full longer.

Diet for off or cardio days

Since the calories on rest days or cardio days are greatly reduced, the eating window is shorter. It works best to have 2-3 good sized meals rather than the 6-7 you read about in muscle magazines. On cardio days, the fast is broken 1 hour after completing the cardio with a 50 g protein shake. Take your first "real" meal two hours after the shake and continue until the 6 hours are up. Carbohydrates are limited to 20 a day and should consist of fibrous green vegetables and trace amounts in foods.

Intermittent Fasting Diet Strength Training Routine

Strength training is a 3-day whole-body routine. Exact days don't matter here either, but make sure you have a day off between workouts. On days 1 and 2, only train the large muscles (legs, back, chest) and add the arms of the smaller muscles/calves) on day 3. You do 4 sets of 6-8 reps for each large muscle and 2-3 sets of 8-12 reps for the smaller ones. Here is an example of a training routine:

Day 1: pushing

Flat bench press / leg press / shoulder press / weighted crunches

Day 2: pull

Rows / Pull-ups / Hamstring Curl

Day 3: push/pull

Bench presses / rows / squats / calf raises / side lifting / barbell curl / triceps pushdown / side lifting / back extensions / weighted crunches

For maximum fat loss, cardio should be lowered 2-3 times a week. Start with a 5-minute warm-up and then start with 10 minutes of High-Intensity Interval Training (HIIT). This works best on an elliptical trainer or a spin bike instead of a treadmill. You will do this at 1-minute intervals. Maximum intensity for 1 minute, followed by a moderate pace for 1 minute. Repeat until 10 minutes have passed. After the HIIT session, drink some water and rest for 5 minutes. After your break, do 30 minutes of cardio with low to medium intensity and stable condition. A treadmill is ideal for this. Don't forget to wait an hour and eat 50g of protein.

Many diets are downright dangerous, especially those where you go to your local pharmacy and buy over-the-counter miracle drugs. The thing they don't tell you is that CHEMICALS ARE UNNATURAL. If you stop taking the pills, the weight will increase immediately. Another thing to remember is that ANY unnatural chemical that is introduced into your body HAS SIDE EFFECTS, it shouldn't be there !!! If you deprive your body of everything it needs, you will not only feel like binge eating in the long run; it will also damage your digestive system and general health. Only grapefruit, only meat, and protein, fad juice diets are further examples of this. Your body needs carbohydrates, just the right ones in the right amounts. Some diets where you need to buy expensive or cheap equipment (as far as that is concerned) while effectively helping to improve muscle tone and not harming your body is damaging your wallet, even with three simple payments. The best way to safely diet is:

1. Easy care without "binge" food.

2. A diet that keeps your body healthy.

3. Introduce exercises that are fun and easy to integrate into your lifestyle.

4. Rewards you with goals and forgives if you slip.

As we get older, our bodies don't have the metabolism we had when we were younger. Sometimes we find ourselves in a position to diet. A better idea is to find a diet that actually represents a lifestyle change. You want to hold the weight, don't you? Be careful out there !! There are many diets that can harm you. If you need to go on a diet, find out how best to diet safely. Basically, the idea behind fasting is to reduce food consumption to bring about weight loss. People associate weight gain with extreme food consumption; Fasting is their way to lose weight quickly. They think that starvation would give them faster results; eventually, lead to weight loss. However, the question remains whether fasting for weight loss is an effective and safe method or not. Obese people have no control over their appetite, which leads to obesity. The idea of fasting is not primarily to lose weight but to gain control over your own appetite. Learning to control the craving for food could lead to weight loss. You limit your food intake during fasting. If you don't eat enough, your body burns fat instead. If you continue, your metabolism will slow down. The body slows it down in response to food restrictions, so you would live longer without food, which is called the survival mechanism. On the lighter side, it cleanses the digestive system and helps to restore and rejuvenate the body. Water makes up most of the solid foods you eat. Fasting will help you lose weight quickly since a large percentage of the weight loss comes from water, but this is only temporary because it does not induce permanent fat loss. In general, effective weight loss should allow the body to burn fat permanently and effectively.

Fasting is undoubtedly not a safe and effective way to lose weight as it can be harmful to your health. It can show a dramatic weight loss to deceive you that it is effective, but the truth is that the loss is only a result of water loss, and fat is quickly restored once you eat. People should learn not to do things easily. There are more effective and safer ways to lose weight, the most common and the most conventional - diet and exercise. Patience and motivation will help you achieve your weight loss goals. Fasting may be the easy way for some, but it does not guarantee a long-term and effective result. Now you want to have greater vigor, be healthier, look younger, lose weight, and clean your body? Intermittent fasting is a controlled fasting pattern that is performed in an alternative manner.

Keys To Understanding Intermittent Fasting

As IF is becoming increasingly popular as a diet for weight loss and health management, it is important to understand how to set it up. Here are three keys to making sure that you can get into an intermittent fasting lifestyle as soon as possible.

- IF does not have to be a short-term approach to dieting and is indeed much more successful as a real lifestyle choice. So the first decision is how to adapt to YOUR life quickly. Remember that fasting can take anywhere from 16 hours to several days, depending on what you want to achieve. The two approaches that are perhaps the easiest to set up are a fast / eat cycle with alternating days (24 hours) or a 16/8 cycle.

- When do you train? This is the key question. Diet is undoubtedly the most important factor in weight loss and good health. However, to get the most out of intermittent fasting, the refill should coincide with your workout. All of the foods you eat during your workout are used as fuel and muscle repair, rather than being filled as body fat.

- What do you want to achieve with intermittent fasting? Is your goal of fat loss, muscle building, improved health, or a combination of all three? In terms of your answer to these questions, you can determine exactly how long you should fast and how much food you should eat during the "meal window."

With intermittent fasting, the eating behavior is switched between fasting periods (water consumption only) and non-fasting (eating). The mealtimes can be very different and extend over several days. Some of the longer non-eating periods include 36-hour fasting followed by 12 hours of eating (usually divided into 3 meals 3-4 hours apart). Most intermittent fasting diets span a 24 hour period so the person can stay constant day by day. The more aggressive of these one-day fasts limits a person to 4 hours of food (usually at night). The most common fasting program includes an 8-hour meal window. Intermittent fasting has been studied extensively in both animals and humans. Unless fasting was extended beyond 36 hours, no negative effects were observed in the test subjects (apart from mild to moderate hunger pains). IF has been shown to reduce body fat, stabilize blood sugar, and increase muscle response. How does it work? It's all about the hormone insulin. Your body releases insulin when you eat food (even more so with carbohydrate foods). Insulin stimulates the absorption of nutrients (mainly glucose) in your fat and muscle tissue. Since energy is not removed from muscle cells most of the time, excess nutrients are stored in your fatty tissue after meals (glucose is also stored as glycogen in your liver). After meals, it takes approximately 3 hours for your body's insulin levels to drop to pre-meal levels. At lower insulin levels, your liver and adipose tissue release the stored glucose and fatty acids into your bloodstream for energy. By increasing the time between meals, you prolong this catabolic state when your body burns fat.

Have you been told to eat 5-6 small meals a day? Frequent consumption of meals actually hinders the body's fat-burning process. On a similar diet, a person who uses an intermittent fasting approach will have a lower body fat percentage than the common eater. However, keep in mind that the quality of your diet is more important than timing. Intermittent fasting is no excuse for eating junk food later that night. You still have to eat clean. You also want to increase your protein intake during a fasting diet. Protein is the best macronutrient in terms of satiety, which means that calorie-by-calorie protein suppresses hunger longer than carbohydrates or fats. A high protein / low carbohydrate diet is a must, especially on days without training. If you don't see any results in your current weight loss program, I strongly recommend you to try the intermittent fasting approach. It takes a week or two before you can fast for 16 hours without feeling extremely hungry. But the results are worth the temporary hunger.

WHAT YOU CAN EAT DURING YOUR INTERMITTENT FASTING

The necessity to eat amino acids during the "fasting state" (especially before and after the morning "fasting state").

Increased need for a delicious, balanced meal when you get out of the fasting state.

This period only lasts for the next 6 to 10 hours, depending on your last meal that day. During this time, it is advisable to eat your 3 main meals. You still have breakfast, also known as (Break the Fast), only at a later time than your normal routine. It doesn't have to include your typical breakfast meal, but it definitely can if that's your thing. Each meal is of a decent size and will keep you strong until the next day. Things to consider during your feeding or fed status:

If you exercise in the evening, try to keep your carbohydrates moderate to low for pre-workout meals and consume a heavy carbohydrate meal after your evening workout to end the day and the resulting feeding condition. Crazy about junk food for your first meal after fasting will completely wipe out all the good that comes from fasting. Let the meals be of normal size and portions. Listen to your body and always wait 15 to 20 minutes after eating to see if you need more food. This is how long it usually takes for a meal to reach your stomach and its sensory receptors that signal hunger.

The reason it is not considered a "diet" is that it does not limit you to certain foods, recipes, combinations, instructions, or tables that you need to follow to lose weight. It frees you from compulsive eating habits and allows you variety. Instead of completely avoiding a particular food because someone has told you, adding a variety of foods prevents you from overeating any type of "bad" food. Example of acceptable foods for the phase 1 diet

1) Eggs

2) FRUIT: berries, grapefruit, lemon, lime, green apples, avocado, fresh

coconut

3) MEAT: Practically all meat, including fish, poultry and beef

4) VEGETABLES: Fresh, immaculate vegetables and freshly prepared vegetable juice

5) DRINKS: Bottled or filtered water, not fruity herbal teas, fresh lemonade sweetened with stevia, freshly squeezed carrot juice.

6) VINEGAR: Apple cider vinegar

7) OILS: olives, grapes, linseed, cold-pressed coconut oil

8) NUTS: raw nuts including pecans, almonds, walnuts, cashews, and pumpkin seeds. Stored nuts tend to collect mold. So be careful!

9) Sweeteners: stevia, xylitol

10) Dairy: organic butter, organic yogurt, (use the following very sparingly) cream cheese, unsweetened whipped cream, real sour cream.

Note: This food selection is only allowed at the beginning of the diet. After a while, you are allowed to introduce more and more types of food, but only when the overgrowth of the mushroom is resolved. There are a couple of phases that he constructed so that you don't have any clue as to what to do next. Keep in mind that the restriction of certain foods only applies for a short time. Starting this diet in conjunction with intermittent fasting will eliminate the guesswork of fat loss. Losing weight is nothing more than burning more calories than you are consuming. Intermittent fasting leads to an enormous calorie deficit.

During fasting, you can and should drink plenty of water to avoid dehydration. Tea and coffee are fine as long as you take just a splash of milk. If you are troubled that you are not getting enough nutrients into your body, consider celery, broccoli, ginger, and lime juice that tastes good and brings some nutrient-rich fluid into your body. If you can do it, it's best to stick to water, tea, and coffee. Whatever your diet is, whether it is healthy or not, you should experience weight loss after about 3 weeks of intermittent fasting and should not be discouraged if you do not notice much progress at first. It is not a race, and it is better to linearly lose weight fashion over time rather than lose a few pounds that you will put on again immediately. After the first month, you may want to take a look at your diet on days without fasting and cut out high-sugar foods and all the trash you normally eat. If you are fasting for bodybuilding at times, you should look at your macronutrients and find out how much protein and carbohydrates you need to eat. Intermittent fasting has many benefits that you will notice as you progress. Some of these benefits include more energy, less bloating, a clearer mind, and general well-being. It is important not to succumb to the temptation to have binge eating after a period of fasting, as this will nullify the effect of intermittent fasting. So if you follow a 24-hour intermittent fasting schedule twice a week for a few weeks, you will lose weight. However, if you can improve your diet on days when you are not fasting, you will lose more weight, and if you can stay with this system, you can reduce weight without resorting to crash diets or diets that you follow just can't hold it.

Advantages And Disadvantages Of Intermittent Fasting With The General Guidelines

Pros:

Create a massive calorie deficit

Increases fat and calorie burning

Increases the ability to recognize true and false feelings of hunger

You don't have to eat every 2-3 hours, which can be a pain in the butt

Increased energy levels and metabolism

Cons:

Women struggle with this diet

Getting used to

You may feel flat at times, but that's not often reported

Guidelines:

It is very different from normal fasting and has many healthy effects on the human body. This method is undoubtedly one of the best ways to lose weight. Wrong fasting is very harmful to your body, but to ensure a good and safe way, intermittent fasting is the way to a healthy lifestyle. Many fitness clinics and nutritionists advocate this method to achieve a healthy lifestyle. Fasting for 2 days (not consecutively) and then eating whatever you want on the other 5 days of the week is a very interesting diet plan for anyone who wants to lose weight and/or live a healthy life. This plan has many advantages. The main benefit of losing weight through this type of fasting is longer life expectancy through a change in diet. With a diet plan, everyone around the world can benefit from intermittent fasting and lose weight. A recent case study showed that people who keep on fasting live about 40% longer than the average lifespan of people in the same country. Moderate fasting protects you from these chronic diseases. Fasting is also a great detoxifier for your body tissues. It is imperative that a diet plan is strictly followed so that your system gets enough rest, and all harmful particles of the body are removed. This process is known as a natural cleansing and restores the natural balance in all major body systems. Improved fitness and weight loss are the two biggest attractions for intermittent fasting. If you follow such a diet, you can achieve your desired body weight. This fasting method is widely used and is a safe and proven method for weight loss. However, if you are pregnant, it should not be used. You will burn all the excess pounds of fat, which will make you physically fitter. Healthy young adults will usually benefit the most from it. It is important that if you think you have a serious health problem, you should see a doctor first to make sure that such a fasting course is safe. Let your body absorb the changes over several steps at a time. This way, you stay fit, healthy, and safe from unwanted effects. Have some amino acids ready and take them in the morning and before/after your workout. Finally, always ask your doctor before trying this.

Intermittent fasting isn't for everyone, but if you're serious about getting real results, it will definitely strengthen you. Everyone should still learn the basics of a healthy diet and exercise program. You can definitely exercise on your fasting days to improve fat loss, but it will be extremely difficult for many to find the energy to do so. Overall, make sure you plan ahead of your fasting day, as this is critical to your success with the program.

HOW TO START?

Before you start fasting, you should consult a professional. However, you can first choose a day on which to skip breakfast. You can choose to drink water or tea instead of breakfast. Later on, try to skip lunch. If you feel like you need to eat something or feel anxious, you can take a full-sized meal. Fasting, by definition, means giving up food and drinks or just eating for a period of time, usually between 8 and 72 hours. Intermittent fasting integrates fasting for 16 to 24 hours into your lifestyle. It can be done daily or several times a week, depending on the length of the fast. It is recommended to start fasting slowly. Initially, you should start with an 18-20 hour fast 1-2 times a week. For example, you can have dinner today at 8 pm and then fast until 2 pm tomorrow afternoon. Drink plenty of water while fasting. You can add some lemon juice or apple cider vinegar to your water. Coffee and tea are fine, too, as mentioned earlier. At 2:00 p.m., you can then break your fast with a normal meal that you would have at this time of day, just in case you had not fasted. Congratulations! You have completed your first intermittent fast! IF is a simple yet effective way to lose fat and especially to get rid of your back fat. The unique option you have to perform is to avoid food for a certain period of time. We recommend starting 1 fast 18 hours a week and then adding a second 18-hour fast in 2-3 weeks.

Our lives are really busy, and our nutrition and energy suffer. In order to maintain a high energy level, discipline is required. The goal of increasing energy naturally offers a solution that takes less time than going to the gym: a healthy lifestyle and a clean mind help to increase your energy. The challenge is to have enough energy to clear the mind. Good habits arise when you pay attention to what your body needs. This article describes ways you can increase your energy without supplements or harmful medication.

Many of the causes of low energy are due to malnutrition. Pay attention to what you eat and naturally increase your energy. Eating right requires knowledge. You need to study what your body requires. If you watch out what you eat, your body will start working with you, not against you. Vitamins help the body function properly. The key is vitamin B. This vitamin correlates directly with the health of your mind. The mind serves the body and energy level. It is crucial that you have enough vitamin B-6 and B-12 to increase energy naturally. The food groups that contain vitamin B-1 are cereals, vegetables, and lean meats. Vitamin B-2 is found in milk, mushrooms, and liver. The last vitamin B-3 that helps you increase your energy is found in bran, chicken, and fish. These aren't the only foods with these vitamins, but it's a start. If you eat more vitamins, you can live a healthier life with more energy.

The increased oxygen level in your blood helps circulate important chemicals in your body. Breathing is essential for you and your body. With a sufficient amount of trace elements of iron and copper in your food, you increase blood circulation and put less strain on your body. If you have balanced iron content in your diet, your system will be balanced. This will remove the effect of fatigue on you. Remember that too much can be harmful to these minerals.

A working mind is essential for a high-energy person. Regular sleep patterns help with this. If you spend many hours awake, you will increase your fatigue for the next day. Because of how a mind works, it uses mental patterns to send messages. These messages are sent as energy waves in the form of a certain frequency. Each frequency vibrates at a different speed. The lower the setting, the more resistance and struggle you will have to keep it going. Many people have a bad attitude when they lack sleep. That is why they work against themselves.

Finally, to increase energy naturally, you need to find and maintain a balance in your life. A balance between nutrition, sleep, and breathing increases your chances of being energized and aware throughout the day. If you ignore these simple steps, you will return to your old patterns. Hear out what your body needs, grow, and enjoy a full life without fatigue.

Before changing your diet, let us point out that this can be a major cause of stress for most people. It will take gradual steps. Don't think it's going to be easy; it won't. But with the right attitude and the right plan, you will definitely see positive changes. Also, discard the setting. It will be difficult". It won't help you. Instead, think of it as a step-by-step process that you incorporate and perform one day after the other. With that said, you can start with the 12/12 split. What does the 12/12 split mean? The 12/12 split simply means that you fast for 12 hours and then eat for the next 12 hours. That means you can start fasting from 7 p.m. to 7 a.m. and eat from 7 p.m. to 7 a.m. The only good thing is that you don't have to adjust your feeding schedule drastically. You may have to postpone breakfast or postpone dinner, but that's all. Very easy and quick to implement. When you start experimenting with the 12/12 split, you may find that you have a bite to eat in the evening. Or that you wake up in the middle of the night to stuff things in your throat. This is simply a case of eating out of habit versus actual hunger. If you create a schedule and stick to it, you will become more aware of your meal times and eating habits.

Start small and give yourself achievable goals. Ensure you know what you're getting into. It's all a mind thing; mental preparation is key. Start small and evaluate your performance as you go. Sign up for an online program to calculate and monitor your calories from your current plan and switch to fewer meals a day (which supports intermittent fasting). Bear in mind that this is a lifestyle change, so it should be based on your lifestyle. Do what makes you comfortable.

Why You Should Try

Intermittent Fasting?

Intermittent fasting is a controversial weight loss technique because it means not eating over a long period of time. Many people have the idea that not eating slows down your metabolism and puts your body in starvation mode, but it turns out this is not true at all. In fact, the human body has been designed to do without food for a long time, so intermittent fasting is a natural practice. Maybe that's why it's so effective. If you want to lose weight but don't want to give up certain foods or don't want to exercise vigorously, intermittent fasting is probably the best option. Fasting helps you lose weight quickly, even if you are not extremely healthy or do not exercise, although this would significantly improve your results. With this technique, you don't even have to lower the number of calories you consume. In the beginning, you just need a little discipline. If you don't like the idea of fasting, the benefits may convince you to try anyway. The results of fasting are affected by exercise volume and other physical activities, recovery ability and patterns, the macronutrient ratios of the diet, the type of exercise program, eating habits and lifestyle, current body composition, and daily lifestyle. That said, you should start with the basic fasting program and monitor your results. Then you can adapt the program to your body needs to maximize the removal of back fat. The results of intermittent fasting are not limited to fat loss. Intermittent fasting can also lead to an increase in muscle mass, health and performance improvements, better digestion of food, and an improved immune function. An important advantage of fasting is the improved insulin resistance, which forms the basis for the fat loss of fasting and the improvement of the metabolism.

For those looking for ways to increase energy naturally, it is a great place to start learning everything you need to know about naturally increasing energy. It is best to first discuss how blood sugar can affect your energy level. Balanced blood sugar is important so that you have enough energy for the day. This does not mean that you should eat a bundle of chocolate or something that is high in sugar. Although this helps increase your energy level, the downside is that your body will eventually crash and feel worse. If you are seeking a way to increase your energy level, you should choose methods that prolong it and not just increase it for a few hours. One of the best methods to increase energy naturally is to include protein in your meals that are mixed with a complex carbohydrate. Protein helps increase your blood sugar, which then helps increase your energy. Chicken, eggs, meat, and fish are good sources of protein. You could have a protein shake for breakfast and then chicken or meet for lunch. End your day with a slice of good meat or fish dinner. This will help you increase your energy in no time. Just be aware that too much protein quickly turns into fat.

Another way to increase your energy is to get enough sleep. This includes a comfortable bed for sleeping so that your body can replenish the energy it lost during the day. Adequate sleep helps restore your body to give you the energy you need for the next day. Adequate sleep is one of the crucial components of a healthy lifestyle. Taking vitamins is also important. There are many supplements to choose from, and it is not difficult to find one that fits your needs perfectly. You may want to seek your doctor, which vitamin supplements can meet your energy needs. This will help you achieve the level of energy that you will have to endure in high spirits in your day.

Diet, proper sleep, and supplements are just a few examples of simple things you can do to improve your lifestyle naturally. There are other methods you can try to increase your energy. Avoid relying on caffeine and sugar products to increase your energy, as it only lasts for a few hours, is unhealthy, and damages your body in the long term. If you want to increase your energy, this is the only way that you can extend your energy throughout the day without harmful side effects. When it comes to how you can naturally increase energy, these methods have been proven to deliver the results you need. There is no doubt that with these steps, you can greet the day with a refreshing and full of life that will help you survive the day with high energy.

Everyone seems to be talking about intermittent fasting these days. Discussions range from incredible to incredulous about the benefits or lack of skipping meals like breakfast. Don't you think breakfast is the healthiest and should be the biggest meal of the day? This leads to the advantages of an intermittent fasting program.

1. Improves immune function (immune system booster)

Human white blood cells are an effective defense mechanism against pathogens in the body. However, white blood cells are limited by their ability to perform their defense functions when entering cells and attacking intercellular pathogens. This is because the primary line of defense of these pathogens is actually lysosomes. Lysosomes through a process known as autophagy, meaning self-eating, act as a cell garbage disposal. Damaged proteins, organelles, viruses, bacteria, and other pathogens are destroyed during autophagy. How long it takes for your last meal to affect lysosomal activity directly. Do you already see the connection? The function of lysosomes is to control the number of nutrients available to the cells for the organelles to use. A filled stomach suppressed the functions of the lysosomes, and therefore no autophagy takes place. Intermittent fasting allows the cells to undergo autophagy, and therefore lysosomes can perform their waste disposal function. Autophagy is important for the destruction of intercellular pathogens by restricting their source of nutrients. Dysfunction of autophagy at the cellular level can lead to all kinds of problems, e.g., certain types of cancer that accelerate the aging process and neurological diseases.

2. Better health

You benefit from better and improved health because a properly functioning immune system offers a more robust defense against pathogens in the body. The only method to stay healthy is to build a strong and robust immune system in your body. Choosing one of the feeding windows for intermittent fasting helps regulate the insulin response and glycemic load on the body. You have heard many, many times, that many lifestyle diseases are the result of too much sugar in the blood. That means the blood sugar level is too high. Diseases such as obesity and diabetes are all associated with it.

3. An excellent way to burn excess fat during exercise

The whole purpose of aerobic endurance training is to burn unwanted fat. Health-conscious gym fans are constantly looking for ways to burn fat. Such intense exercise is a great way to use the body's fat storage instead of using glycogen. By combining intermittent fasting and exercise, you can increase fat utilization through ketosis. This is because your best fat burning exercise is best done when your body is in a state where the glycon is exhausted. I hope these three reasons have been of use to you and will enable you to understand better what this sound about intermittent fasting is about.

How To Make Intermittent Fasting Easier?

The carburetor connection - One of the biggest factors that determine the ease of your fast is the carbohydrate content of the meals that lead to your fasting. I have repeatedly found that high carbohydrate consumption the day before fasting dramatically increases your feeling of hunger and cravings during fasting. The lower your carbohydrate consumption, the easier it seems to be fasting. Fasting is one of the best opportunities to learn the difference between the two since you really get to know the properties of hunger. In any case, hormonal hunger is the result of the interaction of various hormones in your body, regardless of the physiological needs of the body. "Hormonal hunger results from strongly fluctuating insulin levels and is responsible for the strong hunger attacks and wild, irrational cravings that can overwhelm even the most determined dieter. Insulin naturally ebbs and flows in dynamic tension with glucagon. This dynamic tension is maintained for so long insulin levels remain relatively stable, this has not been a problem for most of human existence, but the diet of civilized societies in modern times is a drastic departure from the diet with which mankind has evolved over millions of years. "This is pretty simple since many other hormones play a role in hunger. The important message here, however, is that all hormones play off each other and are triggered by catalysts like the foods you eat. If you have a great attraction for one of your hormones - like throwing sugar at insulin - it is conceivable that you will trigger a cascade cycle of hormonal imbalance that can persist for number of hours (if not days). You can think of it as bringing a wild child into a room with a few calm children. The hooligan will upset the others and excite the whole room. And even if the original wild child gets tired or relaxes, the others will put it back into action. Once you get your hormones up to speed and bounce off each other, it will take a while for them to simmer until hormonal hunger normalizes, and you have a better sense of real hunger. 3 tips to make fasting easier:

1. Don't eat a big meal before you start fasting.

Especially when you start intermittent fasting for the first time, it can be very tempting to stand out before fasting. This is part of the psychological fear of "starvation," a fear that has been intensified by the food industry. But a big meal before fasting will trigger the hormonal imbalance we try to avoid, regardless of the composition of the macronutrients.

2. Avoid sugar before fasting

Of course, I would recommend that you always avoid processed white sugar. But before you fast, you should also consider reducing other sources of simple sugars like dried fruits, high GI fruits like bananas, and milk. All of this will tend to upset your hormones.

3. Avoid starchy carbohydrates

There's nothing wrong with a good sweet potato, a juicy butternut squash, or a nice bowl of steel-cut oatmeal, but before fasting, all of these things could be enough insulin release stimulants to make your hormonal fasting hunger stronger. As for cereals and potatoes, I would try to avoid them most of the time, but I wouldn't wish to touch them with a ten-foot pole before fasting. And of course, all processed food-like substances that are made from white flour should be reduced to a minimum at all times. So what can you eat before your fast? Protein, good fats, and vegetables should be stapled foods. The menu could include beef, chicken, bison, fish, turkey, lamb, broccoli, cauliflower, lettuce, spinach, cucumber, peppers, spring onions, olive oil, coconut oil, etc. Of course, this list is absolutely incomplete, but it is absolutely incomplete gives you the idea. You can fill it in as long as it is similar. Try these three tips, and I'm convinced that your next fast will be a lot easier than one that follows after a high-carb day.

When we eat, the body goes into the digestive mode. Insulin increases because the digestion of the meal produces blood sugar. This takes between 3 and 5 hours. Once you are fed, and the food has been digested, you will be in post-absorbing mode. This means that you are done processing and absorbing nutrients. The insulin has dropped and normalized. You are now in fast mode. The longer you halt here, the more likely your body will burn stored fat for energy. However, if you spend too much time here, your body burns muscles, slows down metabolism, and saves energy. The key is to fast just long enough - and how long it is hotly debated - to burn stored fat and give you the benefits of calorie reduction without the disadvantages mentioned.

The simplest of these plans say that you have to eat within a period of 8 hours - no matter which 8 hours - and for 16 quickly. It might look like having dinner at 8 a.m., skipping breakfast, and eating again at 1 a.m. Yes, for some. For hypoglycemia, this is not a plan for you. For others, the body adapts, you do not die, the consequences for those who want to lose weight can blow a traditional diet out of the window. Why is it mainly because it's easier to limit meal times than how much or what you eat. If IF is a good idea or you just want to try it out to see how you feel and if you lose weight, start by shortening the hours on the day you eat. IF falls into the category of calorie reduction, which science has researched well as a way to extend lifespan. Animal studies have supported and warned IF as a bridge to more health and longevity. Scientific America has published a comprehensive article on this. We are in the early stages of IF science, but it is hard not to believe in the science that exists. If you try, monitor how you feel when you fast. Do not walk longer than it feels safe, but be ready to feel hungry. Learning to feel real hunger against the urge to eat out of boredom or fear is one of the advantages of IF. Now that I am no longer forced to follow someone else's rules, when I eat or why I will experiment with IF without feeling guilty or thinking for a minute that it will be my salvation.

Weekly Diet Plan

It seems everyone is on a diet, and rightly so since the majority of people are obese. How come? Can anything be done to get the nation back in shape and set up a weekly diet plan? There is a possibility that no one has heard of intermittent fasting as a means of burning fat, but of fasting for religious purposes. Many religions include compulsory fasting as a way to purify the body spiritually, like the Islamic religion and its month of Ramadan. But can fasting be used to cleanse the body while losing weight? It certainly can, and lately, people have used this method to cut unwanted inches on their bellies and waists. Many people are against fasting because they believe they have to eat constantly to maintain their metabolism. That is simply not true. Clinical studies have found that the body's metabolism is directly related to the amount of lean body mass or muscles in the individual. Those with less muscle have slower metabolism compared to those who are more muscular. It has nothing to do with the frequency or amount of meals, as food companies want the general public to believe. Here are some action lines to keep in mind when fasting:

Fasting on non-consecutive days. So if you fast at times on Monday, try not to fast again until Wednesday

Don't fill up after fasting (you'll be tempted to overeat, but not)

Do not eat excessively sugary foods if you are going away from fasting

Drink enough water while fasting (especially if you get hungry, it helps to drink extra water)

Coffee helps curb appetite. So drink a cup of "Joe" on the morning of your fast, but don't add sugar as this will break the fast. Bonus: Apply stevia in your coffee as a sweetener.

The bonuses for following your weekly diet plan and adding intermittent fasting are numerous. First of all, you save on food costs. Since you eat less, there are fewer trips to the grocery or restaurant. Second, you don't have to think about or prepare what you will eat that day. Our lives are constantly asking ourselves, " In addition, by adding IF to your eating plan, you can finally control the urge to eat, which is half the battle for trying to lose pounds and inches. IF should be an integral part of your weekly diet plan if it has not already done so. There is no better way than IF to reduce calories and achieve tremendous health benefits easily.

How do you get slim?

Perhaps you've heard the advice to eat a few small meals throughout the day to reduce fat and keep blood sugar constant. However, scientific studies on intermittent fasting have shown that it itself has some very impressive health effects. It improves insulin sensitivity so that there are no spikes in blood sugar, and lowers blood pressure, heart rate and protects against oxidative stress. These studies even showed an extended lifespan and reduced cancer incidence. All of these advantages come to slim down. With fasting, you lose healthily and not only for a limited period of time but consistently lead to a permanently slim body! So ... why use fasting for weight loss? There are various methods of weight loss and literally thousands of programs to choose from. So you may be wondering why you should choose fasting rather than dieting. The mere mention of fasting may sound daunting for many.

Before you get caught up in the idea of fasting, however, you need to understand what fasting really means and how it can help reduce stubborn excess weight. First of all, it is necessary to understand that the type of fasting to consider is not the type that you imagine in your head. Fasting or intermittent fasting is an increasingly common way of fasting. Once you know how to incorporate it into your lifestyle, you will lose weight easily and healthy. When done correctly, you can see directly how intermittent fasting works and ultimately have lifelong consequences.

For intermittent fasting to work for you, you should first assess your diet and eating habits. You need to find out what's wrong with the food you eat and how to eat it so you can start making healthy dietary changes. The next thing you need to learn is how to cope with your appetite. Most people who are constantly struggling with obesity have lost control of their craving for food. Short-term or intermittent fasting trains your body so that you can tell the difference between cravings and real hunger. When your body gets habituated to intermittent fasting, you can incorporate healthy dietary changes into your lifestyle. Over time, as healthy eating and regular fasting become routine and, therefore, much easier to manage; you will find that it will be amazingly easy to keep your weight at the desired or recommended level.

Glucose, glycogen, and fat

Your body needs the energy to run properly, and it gets that energy from the food you eat. Food becomes a sugar form called glucose. Your cells (and particularly those in your brain) require a constant supply of glucose. When it gets low, you feel tired and weak. Glucose circulates in your blood after eating and is consumed fairly quickly in your daily chores. If it is not refilled, it will actually be used up in a few hours. This creates a problem: how do you maintain good care? Glucose itself cannot be stored, but it can be converted to a form called glycogen, which can be retained in your muscles and liver. From here, it can be pulled out and used as needed. It is usually good for around 10 to 12 hours. What happens when it is exhausted? The body turns into fat cells stored in the body. They are broken down and converted into so-called ketones. Of course, this is what dieters are looking for: fat cell loss. However, be careful if you stay in this phase for a long time. The body immediately begins to break down proteins. It can be converted to glucose in a rather complex process. And that leads to muscle loss - something you don't want. In fact, with most diets, a fair amount of weight loss comes from muscle loss along with water shortage (which makes you dehydrated). So don't be fooled.

One of the hormones in your body is called IGF-1 (insulin-like growth factor 1); It helps your cells grow and is especially important in growing children. However, when you reach adulthood, it decreases significantly. This is important as it appears to have adverse effects with increasing age: it accelerates aging and can even lead to cancer. So it's not something you want when you are older. And studies have shown that intermittent fasting reduces it. There is also a protein in your brain called BDNF (brain-derived neurotrophic factor). It is important because it has been shown to help stem cells transform into new neurons. This happens in a section of the brain, the hippocampus, which is vital for memory and learning. BDNF has many effects: it seems to protect against dementia and Alzheimer's and also acts as an antidepressant and suppresses anxiety. Finally, intermittent fasting also helps to increase autophagy. This is a system in the cells that removes damaged molecules that can lead to serious neurological diseases.

Diabetes comes in two forms: Diabetes I and Diabetes II. We will mainly deal with Diabetes II. As we saw earlier, all cells use glucose as fuel. But without insulin, it cannot get into the cells. Insulin is produced in the pancreas according to the amount of glucose in the blood; Your job is to get the glucose into the cell. Most cells in your body have so-called insulin receptors, which bind to the insulin that circulates in your blood. When a cell has insulin partial to its surface, it lets the glucose in, so it obviously plays an important role in your body. But too much can be harmful. Insulin increases your hunger, promotes the storage of fat cells, and has been linked to diabetes and heart problems. One of the main problems with insulin is the so-called insulin resistance. In this case, the pancreas produces insulin, but the insulin receptors in the cells no longer work properly and do not let the glucose enter as it should. Without space, the glucose continues to circulate in the blood, and the cells soon begin to starve. The body recognizes that something is wrong, and the pancreas produces more insulin to bring sucrose into the cells. However, this leads to an overload of the pancreas and eventually begins to wear out. The result is Diabetes II. Studies have shown that IF improves insulin sensitivity. This, in turn, allows your body to control your blood sugar levels after meals better, helping to rest your pancreas. Both are important for the prevention of diabetes II.

Fasting rules

It is best to use a 5-2 approach, with regular meals 5 days a week and two days with restricted food (500 calories for women, 600 for men). Drink enough. Drink plenty of water; It helps flush out toxins. If you are not on fasting days (and even during fasting), keep your diet maximized. In particular, eat enough vegetables, fruits, and whole grains. Remember that the effect requires 12 hours of fasting. 12 to 18 hours is best. The plateau is beyond 18. You can exercise during Lent, but don't overdo it. Be careful when fasting if you are diabetic.

IMPACT OF INTERMITTENT FASTING

What is IF, and why should you care? Intermittent fasting has become very popular in circles in which people are looking for ways to reduce calorie intake without affecting their exercise goals, but which still allow them to lose weight during weight training. Intermittent fasting is the practice of short-term fasting, 24 hours, once or twice a week. There are variations on this topic, but in general, this is the norm. This is not done as much to "cleanse" the system as many would think, although to some extent it will. It's just a simple and quick way to reduce calorie intake so you can achieve your weight loss goals without hunger plans or other diets. You don't have to be overanxious about the types of foods you consume while not fasting, although note that fasting once or twice a week doesn't really help you achieve your goals if you expend the other five or six days in which you stuff yourself with all kinds of garbage. A little common sense is required.

By allowing reasonable freedom in your food choices, it relieves the anxiety that most diets have. We often feel totally constrained and restricted, while this approach allows us not only to choose what we want to consume but also to bring balance and sanity back into our diet. Intermittent fasting as a lifestyle leads to changes that last a lifetime. First, take it slowly and really learn to listen to what your body tries to tell you as you endure your first few weeks. If you feel lethargic or malnourished, change it a little. Your body will let you know what it needs. (And that's usually not a monster double cheeseburger!) Often, especially in the beginning, your body will go through some draws, and it's important to learn how to distinguish the signals. You also need to consider the impact of exercise routines that you are involved in on your intermittent fasting plans. The most important thing about intermittent fasting is that it is not just a diet plan but a lifestyle that should be considered in this sense. To get the best possible results from this type of plan, you need to befriend it. Your fasting should be something you look forward to, as you will for sure when you start to take advantage of some of the benefits of this intermittent fasting. Integrating this type of plan into your life is key to enabling good food and healthy living for a lifetime. There is a lot of freedom in such a diet plan, and if you are not careful, it can lead to failure, but it can also lead to lasting success. See what intermittent fasting can do for you!

Intermittent fasting may seem like a catastrophic technique to lose weight by starving your body, but in reality, it is not true. As the name suggests, it is an irregular hunger, not a normal one, so the routine is more useful than harmful. You don't have to eat sporadically, but vice versa. This means that a person can continue their usual eating routine without having to do anything about calorie intake. So if the diet consists of bacon and eggs in the morning, a subway sandwich in the afternoon, and a portion of lasagna in the evening, this eating pattern doesn't have to break. The only difference that is observed is a 24-hour pause during which the item to be consumed is water. This fasting is more or less like giving the digestive system a break from fats, carbohydrates, and proteins. The idea is not to overwork the body if it eats too much food, and less time to break it down through aerobic and anaerobic exercises, but to give the inner system a break. The best thing about this "rest," however, is that during this period, the metabolism is accelerated, and all impurities are removed as the only main consumption is water.

In fact, it is not just the hunger of a day that does the magic, but rather the consumption of water that increases the results. The advantages of water have always been demonstrated. For every illness, the doctor emphasizes the absorption of water. Beauticians emphasize the importance of water to keep the skin free of acne and to keep it glowing. Dietitians emphasize water intake. Even with aerobic and anaerobic exercises, it is emphasized again and again how important good water intake is. What magic does water actually have on the body, making it act like such a reliable ingredient? As mentioned above, water speeds up the body's metabolism. Since the kidneys need water to function properly and most people out there absorb little water, it is up to the liver to make up for the loss of water. This lowers overall liver performance or productivity. Since, among other functions of the liver, the main function is to metabolize the stored fat, the liver cannot metabolize the fat after performing the functions for the kidney, which leads to an increase in the extra pounds that accumulate on the figure.

The intermittent fasting period of 24 hours, which can be up to 36 hours depending on the person's will, is a day on which the liver can perform its functions without having to make a contribution due to the lack of kidney functions in the Water Body. This way, the body works more on the stored fats and burns them effectively. So the rest of the day of nutrition is primarily a day to boost metabolism and break down all the extra fat that the body has consumed due to the lack of enough water. Another advantage that intermittent fasting has for the body, in addition to accelerating the metabolism, is the possibility of losing all of the water weight stored in the body. How the water was stored in the hips, thighs, legs, and stomach is mainly due to inconsistent water flow. The body stored all of the water because it did not receive the required amount every day. As soon as the water supply is sufficient, the body automatically decides to let go of all the water stored in the form of fat and drastically reduces body weight. In addition, it has been observed that the body needs less food when there is plenty of water. During the intermittent fasting period, when the body consumes a large amount of water, there is less desire for food because the stomach appears to be well fed. Accordingly, water also helps to maintain muscle mass, which enables better training. So if you want to walk for 45 minutes during your intermittent fasting or get up on the treadmill, the most important solution is to keep yourself fresh after your workout to keep yourself well hydrated. Intermittent fasting is indeed the best way to work towards a consistent weight loss program. However, the results will not be immediate, but there will not be a period of even a week in which a 1 pound loss is not shown on the scale. Accepting this ritual is an intelligent technique for intelligent weight loss.

Intermittent fasting is a method that, when used correctly, can significantly improve your health and increase your weight loss. "Fasting" is a term employed to describe a period in which you can do without food, as is common in some religious practices. The term "intermittent" refers to the alternation of eating and fasting periods. So intermittent fasting is basically a practice of eating within a certain time frame and fasting before and after. We all do this every day since we don't eat in our sleep, but most of us don't "fast" long enough to take advantage of it. Let us discuss how you can change your way of eating so that you can lose weight extremely easily without changing the type of food you eat or the number of calories you eat. To get the most out of IF, you need to fast for at least 16 hours. From 16 hours, some of the amazing benefits of intermittent fasting come into effect. An easy way to do this is to skip breakfast every morning. This is actually very healthy, but a lot of people will try to tell you otherwise. If you skip breakfast, you can allow your body to have a calorie deficit that significantly accentuates the amount of fat you can burn and the weight you can lose. Since your body is not busy digesting the foods you eat, it has time to focus on burning your fat reserves for energy and cleaning and detoxifying your body. If you have difficulty skipping breakfast, you can skip dinner instead, although it is much more difficult. It really doesn't matter, but the goal is to extend the time you spend fasting and shorten the time you spend eating. If you have dinner in the evening at 6 a.m. and do not eat until 10 a.m. the next morning, you have fasted for 16 hours. Longer is better, but you can see some pretty drastic changes from a 16-hour fast every day. There are many ways to fast, and it is important that you choose the path that best suits your lifestyle so that you can stick to it and make it a lifelong habit.

How Can You Apply Intermittent Fasting To Your Life?

Losing weight is something that many people all over the world face. However, what most people don't realize is that intermittent fasting is the best approach that you can really lose weight if you're having trouble losing those extra pounds. Losing weight is not and should not be difficult. People make a big deal out of something that should be a slow and fun process that everyone can enjoy. Intermittent fasting and fasting, in general, is known all over the world, which is very good for health. But people, in general, don't want to go anywhere near it. People think that fasting is something people struggle with, but the great thing about intermittent fasting is that you only do it occasionally. Also, a day that you fast from time to time is a great way to overcome the plateau that you may have reached by losing the excess weight that you have on yourself. The best way to apply intermittent fasting to your life is to start slowly and gradually increase the time you do it. This way, you can get your body used to the whole process and see the results without overwhelming yourself. So the key is to start slowly and slowly increase the time you spend. Make sure you don't do it more than once a week for maximum benefits.

Another thing to remember is that intermittent fasting isn't the only thing you need to do to lose weight effectively. This must be part of a large program that you will be using to live a healthier life. You have to ensure that your diet is perfect, and you have to make sure that you implement an appropriate exercise routine in your life. Only when these things are perfect will you find that you will see the long-term results you are looking for. Intermittent fasting is not an end in itself, but something that must be part of a larger strategy. This is the only method to be successful. It's best to choose a day you work instead of fasting on the weekend. You have a lot to do at work, and that distracts you from eating. You will also find that you have more energy when fasting because your body is not focused on digesting food - this means that you are doing more. You may not need special fasting foods, just make sure you drink plenty of water. If you stay hydrated and busy, your fasting day will pass very quickly, and you will not miss not eating

Don't be too fast or too short-the ideal speed of weight loss and health benefits is 16 to 24 hours, depending on age, experience, and precise goals. Less than this will not really give you the results you want (remember that you are already fasting 10-12 hours overnight), and longer than this is simply unnecessary and can be more difficult to adjust.

Increase your water intake while fasting - Intermittent fasting also helps cleanse your system and make your body work more efficiently. To support this process, you should increase your water intake. The best solution to do this is to always have a glass/bottle of water with you so that you can drink a sip regularly.

Break your fast with a healthy meal - The first thing you eat after a fat should be a healthy meal. Aside from the obvious benefits of a healthy diet, there is less room for junk. Given that you may only have 8 hours to eat your daily meal, it's always a good option to top up the good stuff first.

Time your food around your workout - It goes without saying that training should be part of a healthy eating plan. The heart of your training efforts should be weight training or bodyweight training. Try to eat most of your food immediately after your workout. Thereby, your body will use these calories for reconstruction and repair rather than being stored as fat.

Don't sweat the details - One of the real benefits of intermittent fasting is that there is no demand to count calories or grams of macronutrients. This can be painful and makes dieting difficult. Follow the principles and the details will take care of themselves.

Intermittent Fasting - What Is It, And How Does It Work?

Intermittent fasting is becoming increasingly popular for losing fat, toning, and improving health. But what are the principles behind this approach, and what are the advantages? Fasting is always without food. This can range from a few hours (think sleep, for example) to a few days. While such programs are based on one or more 24-hour fasts per week, this is not the only way to constitute fasting. Here we come to one of the real advantages of this diet over other possible diets. It can be adapted to your life instead of forcing yourself on you and forcing you to adapt to it if a 24-hour cycle suits you, great. If not, a 16 or 20-hour cycle may work better. Does fasting mean that nothing can be absorbed? The answer here is clearly no. The advantage of fasting is that it can "reset" your body so that it can cleanse itself. This is difficult if the digestive tract is permanently burdened by constant digestion. Drinking more water and green tea during this time can help and speed up the cleaning process. Perhaps the most underestimated aspect of intermittent fasting is its impact on the amount of food we eat. Instead of grazing all day every day (a completely unnatural way to eat), a period without food automatically reduces calorie intake and gives you the satisfaction of not being hungry all the time, as is the case with most low-calorie diets. But what about health? Without going into science, there are some obvious health benefits here. One example is fat loss and especially the dangerous belly fat "heart attack." Improved digestive function is another.

With an intermittent fasting diet, however, consumers can eat whatever their heart desires for a full day or twenty-four hours. The food consists of all sorts of ingredients that you would normally consume, dairy products, fats, and anything else you could wish for. But it's the type of fast that actually allows your metabolism to burn it the next day, which is fast. So the principle is simple: from eating to fasting and over and over again, without skipping everyone. For some, this seems to be an extremely simple solution, while others can easily starve to death instead of eating normally for an entire day. During your fasting period, the ingredients ingested are evenly distributed throughout the body, giving you enough strength to deal with the fasting. In the next twenty-four hours, eat and prepare for another fast! This cyclical intermittent fasting diet can actually be very attractive to people who really like to eat, but on the other hand, it has proven effective, which is even more amazing.

The most important fact is that this diet has proven itself several times when losing weight without harming our organism - on the contrary. The fast days allow our metabolism to work pretty busily as there is enough to burn in our body due to the previous "eating" day! The important thing is that the metabolism does not slow down because "it knows" that we are feeding it another day, and the cycle is repeated, which only makes us burn faster - which is actually perfect and healthy to win! Many people are beginning to see the link between fasting and weight loss and are experiencing all the benefits of healthy and natural weight loss. Intermittent fasting is even said to help you live longer because it improves insulin resistance. Insulin resistance is the largest catalyst for many health factors, including weight loss and muscle building, anti-aging, and disease prevention.

The process involves developing an eating cycle that follows an "eat, stop, eat" approach. Basically, you can (seriously) eat whatever you want in the first 24 hours, followed by a period of fasting that should cover the next 24 hours without forgetting to learn the basics like water. Then simply repeat the cycle. This was a more natural way of eating, probably the way cavemen eat. Consider-if you catch an animal one day, they will probably eat a big meal, followed by a period of "downtime" before the next hunt is possible. In the meantime, they have prepared their natural defenses for periods of hunger and increased their metabolism to give them the energy to search for their food. That's how the body protects itself.

Fourteen amazing truths about intermittent fasting

1. You won't feel nearly as hungry as you think.

2. Your concentration will improve dramatically.

3. You save money. It's really an obvious benefit - you don't pay for foods you don't eat.

4. The weight will drop from you like crazy. I was amazed at how quickly the excess pounds were taken off and keep walking. Losing weight quickly is a formality.

5. You will feel happier. You are on your way to the body you deserve, and every week shows you the progress you are making. It's really motivating and empowering.

6. Nothing in your life needs to be changed.

7. You have more time.

8. Great sleep.

9. Much more energy.

10. Compulsive eating is massively reduced.

11. You can make it part of your life overnight.

12. No tiny ready meals or snack bars.

13. Eat whenever you want. No breakfast? Do not worry. It's overrated anyway. Don't you want to eat little and often? No problem. Just eat as you normally would and fast one or two 24-hour fasts a week.

14. Gain trust. When you get leaner, and your clothes fit better - and buy new ones - you can't help but feel more confident. It is a good feeling!

CONCLUSION

Is it just a flash in the pan, or is it here to stay? Intermittent fasting seems to have come out of nowhere in the past few months. Intermittent fasting, which is actually a rather fancy (sometimes daunting) phrase for two windows - one window when you eat and one window when you don't eat. Intermittent fasting and bodybuilding can work for you if your goal is to build muscle and get lean. A recent study has shown that it is actually the total macros and the total amount of daily calories that are responsible for muscle growth and not the amount and timing of meals. Essentially, this means that it doesn't matter when you get the calories, as long as you get the required amount of calories within 24 hours. As long as you get the required amount of calories (an excess of your TDEE is needed in combination with a progressive workout routine) in your eating window, you will build muscle. One facet of intermittent fasting bodybuilding that people complain about is the amount of food and calories that must be consumed within the window consumed. Although you will most likely need to adjust if you are currently eating 6-8 small meals a day, your stomach will adapt to larger meals over a period of a few weeks. Take time to adjust and don't expect to be able to switch overnight. Remember, like everything else, that intermittent fasting is not an exact science. If you need to expand our meal window from an eight-hour meal window to a nine-hour window to cover all of your calorie and food needs, that's fine. As with any program, it is important to find what works for you. Intermittent fasting, bodybuilding, and muscle building can work together. The nice thing is that when you find the sweet spot that's right for you, you can take advantage of intermittent fasting while keeping or building your body to a bodybuilding level.

With so many food trends, it's difficult to determine which to try. Many users spend more time with the yo-yo than we actually regain most of the weight, counteracting our desired results. Fasting may or may not be tried by many of us. When we try this type of diet, we usually don't do it properly or get frustrated by the restrictions we give up. In the end, we feel like we've wasted our time, effort, and energy just to end up with the results empty-handed. Intermittent fasting is not something that many have heard of. This is due to the fact that it is a fairly new way to eat. This new form of eating will soon provide the nation with benefits that we could all enjoy. With this diet, you can expect to not only lose weight but possibly live longer. If this diet is carried out correctly, your body may be better equipped to deal with the health conditions it may or may not be exposed to in the future. This diet is very simple, but the rewards are nothing more than. You will lose weight, burn that stubborn fat, build muscle, and even increase your growth hormone. Why not give it a try after all the time you've spent with the yo-yo? There are no restrictions on what you can eat during the intermittent fasting diet. Yes, grab the greasy hamburger or the french fries.

You are limited to the periods between eating and fasting. For the first twenty-four hours, you are let go to eat so much and want your favorite things. However, the next twenty-four hours consist of water only. You are probably so full that you want nothing more than water anyway. Continue this cycle, and that's it. This diet stop-eat method of dieting is sure to work for you. You will lose fat with this diet, but not because you eat less. You actually consume about as many calories as if you hadn't fasted with water on the second day. This process gives you the best of both worlds. You can still eat all of your favorites while losing the weight you want. Introducing intermittent fasting into your lifestyle should be fairly easy if you already have pretty good eating habits. The only difference is that you don't eat for a few days. You can continue to operate your business as usual and still benefit from the advantages. For years, doctors and scientists have agreed that the only true form of weight management is calorie reduction. Calorie reduction works for you every time you are able to stick to it. Most people who try low-calorie diets often fall off the car because they are constantly hungry. Despite the fact that you eat reduced calories every day, you usually don't care what you eat. However, with intermittent fasting, you are in control of what you eat and are satisfied when you leave the dining table. If you don't feel like you're on a diet, stick to it.

One very important thing about fasting is that while you can get away with less optimal eating habits than with a normal diet, the food quality makes fasting much easier. You can actually gain weight when fasting if you eat sugary processed foods during your mealtime instead of focusing on quality meats, vegetables, nuts, seeds, and fruits. In the end, there is no "best" way. The best way is what easily fits into your lifestyle and allows you to focus on life, not when your next meal is coming.

Generally, fasting involves self-deprivation of food, liquids, or both. On the other hand, fasting can be done in different ways, e.g., only with water, fasting with fruit or vegetable juice, with interruptions, etc. In many cases, however, the individual will completely refrain from eating. Unfortunately, when talking about achieving fast weight loss goals, the answer to the question is fast, not as cut and dry as many would hope, since the answer is both yes and no! As with everything else in life, most things are okay in moderation, and fasting is no different. If you fast for too long, the effects can be negative, causing diseases and conditions ranging from anorexia to liver failure. Fasting for a comparatively short period of time, but regular, can offer many benefits, including gut health and clearer skin, as well as weight loss. While it is 100% true that the many types of fasting help people lose weight fairly quickly, it can also be true that much of that weight is made up of liquids and not fat, at least initially anyway and only when You would be It means that you do not consume any water or food, which, by the way, is not recommended!

Fasting slows down your metabolism. - This means that the fat you want to lose burns much more slowly, so you won't lose any more weight. This is true, but what is not highlighted is how long you need to be sober for your metabolism to slow down. Think of it this way, most of us have done a diet or two, but what all diets do, regardless of how they are disguised, is to reduce their daily calorie intake. What we find with all diets is that they all reach a weight loss plateau, most are around the two-week mark. This plateau is when the weight loss you have experienced with the diet in the past two weeks is either slowing down drastically or stopping completely! The reason for this is that the body's metabolism has adapted to the new lower calorie intake, and as soon as it does, it stops burning the fat reserves. Fasting for a long time has the same effects; it also reaches a plateau. However, intermittent fasting periods of 24 hours have no effect on your metabolism, but they do reduce your weekly calorie intake.

Fasting is not recommended for people with health problems. - If a person has an existing health problem or is taking certain medications, fasting should be avoided because fasting can easily worsen these health conditions or affect the immune system. An unhealthy person needs all the nutrients they can get, while every person taking certain medications needs significant digestive materials to safely take those medications and even help them take their intended actions. Most of it is true, but many diseases would benefit greatly from intermittent fasting, and there are alternative medications for most ailments that work just as well without food as with food. Always remember, we're talking about intermittent fasting periods of no more than 24 hours, a third of which is spent on sleep! I am sure there are many millions of Muslims and people of other religions who often fast for religious reasons and, at the same time, take and fast take medication safely. It is safest always to consult your doctor.

Ultimately, the problem of fasting safety depends entirely on the circumstances. There are certain critical factors that, if ignored, can pose a real health hazard. However, follow a sensible fasting policy created by nutritionists who base their work on scientifically proven facts. The road to safe, natural weight loss is open.

www.ingramcontent.com/pod-product-compliance
Lightning Source LLC
Chambersburg PA
CBHW031213160726
47992CB00006B/2719